# You are you

love + hugs,
Annabelle xxxx

You are You



Any medical information in this book is based on the author's personal experience and should not be relied on as a substitute for professional advice.

ISBN 978-1-905912-78-0

**I am dedicating this book to all those I love.**

Follow Annabelle on socials

Instagram @annabelletalks

YouTube AnnabelleTalks

CONTENTS

**Introduction** 7

**Chapter One: Girl Talk** 11
Starting Puberty 13
PMS (Premenstrual Syndrome) 16
Menstrual Cycle Phases 23
Periods 29
Toxic Shock Syndrome 61
Irregular Periods 65
My Period Story 68
Endometriosis 77
Fear of the Smear 82
Vaginal Discharge 84
Body Hair 87
Weight Change 89
Bras 92
Skin 95

**Chapter Two: Confidence** 101
Love Your Body 103
Influence of Social Media 117
Feeling Shy 121
Bullying 125

**Chapter Three: Mental Health** **129**
Anxiety 132
Depression 141
Working Out for Your Mental Health 144
Trauma 149
Dealing With Loss 153
Inner Critic 156
Be Kind to Yourself 159

**Chapter Four: Happiness** **163**
Your Personal Space 165
Internet Detox 166
Health 171
Therapy 173
Meditation 176
Mindfulness 182
Journaling 184
Gratitude 188
Manifesting 191
Forward Planning 194
Habits 196
Sleep 206
Self-Care 214
Self-Love 218
**My Thoughts Journal** **221**

# INTRODUCTION

I have written this book to share my personal life. The truth, no secrets, just me.

Some things in my life may have caused me heartache and were painful, but I have learnt so much from my past, and realised that you can bring out the positives in any situation. It is entirely up to you what you take from my stories, but even if you change one tiny thing in your life for the better, I am happy and proud of you.

I am not a doctor, a therapist or any professional coach, I am simply someone who likes to learn and share my experiences with others. I have realised that the good and the bad are both parts of who I have become as a person, and that working on yourself should be the most important thing in life.

Make sure you become better than the person you were yesterday in each and every way, for the rest of your life. Stop trying to impress people. Impress yourself and be the best version of yourself that you can be.

I believe we are all here to make a difference in other people's lives, and I hope that by sharing what is in this book, I can make a difference to yours.

So, just before we get onto the book, I thought I would share a few facts about myself so that you can get to know me a little:

- I love popcorn
- I love travelling to new places and experiencing different cultures
- I love anything that gets my creative juices flowing
- I love sushi and pizza, although not together
- I love antiques and anything sentimental
- I am a good listener, however, I do also love to talk

... and I love helping people in any way that I can.

It is now time to focus on you. I hope you enjoy the book and would love to hear your thoughts.

Regardless of your skin colour, body shape or weight, you are beautiful and this book is written for you.

YOU ARE YOU.

Love and hugs, Annabelle xxxx

# Girl Talk

"THAT'S THE REAL TROUBLE WITH THE WORLD. TOO MANY PEOPLE GROW UP"

– *Walt Disney*

## STARTING PUBERTY

This is the time in your life when your body changes and you become capable of reproduction or having babies. This process typically happens between the ages of 10 and 15 but is different for everyone, so do not worry if you are before or after your friends, as I was about 15 when I started my periods, and there is no shame in this. The main hormonal changes in puberty are the levels of oestrogen and progesterone. Did you know your ovaries since birth have contained millions of little eggs, but it is only when puberty starts and changes happen, that those eggs start maturing? This then means your body is ready for your period to start.

How will my body change?

For us girls, puberty includes an increase in height, a widening of hips, pubic hair, as well as leg and armpit hair, periods, boobs, and spots. You may also notice you start to sweat more and develop your very own body odour - how wonderful.

As you go through puberty, you may also experience all or some of the below changes.

- Curlier and more coarse pubic hair
- Hair in other places such as on your face, perhaps on your upper lip
- Boobs increasing in size
- Acne and spots depending on your own body and hormones
- Vaginal discharge

- An increase in weight as your body changes
- Mood changes

After a few more years your body may change again slightly. Your boobs will become fuller and more adult-like, and your pubic hair may be a little wider spread. You will also have reached your full height and your body will be fully developed, meaning your hormones should balance themselves out a little more and fluctuate less.

## PMS

PMS stands for premenstrual syndrome. This is something most girls will experience 1-14 days before their period. Each of us will go through different symptoms, so it is totally and completely normal if yours differ from your friends'. This is because of how our bodies react differently to our own hormones.

Our lifestyle choices may also affect our menstrual cycle. Have you noticed that in those months where you have eaten better and exercised more, your periods have also been better? I notice a massive difference with mine, even if I choose to just exercise the week before my period and nothing else. Now when it comes to PMS symptoms, like I said above it differs for us all, but most girls will have at least one symptom. Do not panic though as these are usually not severe enough to affect your daily life.

Headaches/Migraines

Hormone levels changing can cause headaches. Personally, I am very prone to them throughout the month, but a few days before my period and a couple of days in, I often experience horrendous headaches as well as migraines. This is completely normal due to hormone imbalance, but if you are struggling, your doctor may prescribe you some hormone replacement tablets to help balance your levels a little.

Relieve those menstrual headaches

- Drink plenty of water
- Eat nuts and lean protein

- Drink grape juice
- Take Vitamin E supplements
- Take Paracetamol

Sore boobs

Your boobs may feel slightly sore to touch, and they can often feel larger too in the lead up to your period. If you have larger boobs this may cause a bit of discomfort when exercising, but I would personally just use that as an excuse to have a day off.

Menstrual cramps

This is pain around your lower tummy area, as well as your lower back on the first couple of days of your period, but unfortunately you may experience pain up to 14 days before your period too. This should not be anything major and continuous, but some pains are normal. I tend to start experiencing cramps around 3 days before my period, which I do find rather handy actually, in case I forget to check my calendar or period tracker app, as it then gives me a few days to prepare myself.

Spots

Those little terrors that seem to just appear without reason? These are hormonal spots and will tend to be around your chin and forehead, frustrating I know.

Cravings

Chocolate, chocolate, and more chocolate. I have not ever been a huge chocolate fan, so as soon as I crave a chocolate bar I know my period is due. Chocolate is the most common craving, but it could be anything. I attempt (emphasis on this word) to eat healthy balanced meals throughout the month so that when it comes to cravings just before my period, I can indulge a little, and not feel too guilty.

Bowel changes

This unfortunately is one of the more unpleasant symptoms, but constipation and diarrhoea are common. I tend to experience constipation a couple of days before my period, and then often have loose stools during the first couple of days.

Bloating

Sadly, being a girl means bloating is part of the package. Certain foods will cause flare-ups, but again we are all different, so it is just a matter of finding out what works for you. Carbohydrates such as pasta and bread seem to be the biggest causes of bloating for me, and this is rather common. Menstruation is also a huge factor to bear in mind as your period makes you retain fluid. Drinking as much water as possible during this time is recommended, as well as avoiding processed food, as salt adds to water retention.

## Emotions

You may find yourself overly happy one minute and crying the next, and this again is totally normal. The week before my period, my emotions seem to be extremely heightened and even happy movies make me cry. Days also feel so much longer due to tiredness, and you may find you are feeling exhausted even if you have not done much. Your body is using a lot of energy preparing for your period so it is normal to feel this way.

If PMS symptoms affect your daily lifestyle there are a few things that might help:

- Regular exercise
- Do not smoke
- Reduce alcohol intake (if you drink)
- Manage your stress levels
- Focus on getting enough sleep
- Remain hydrated

## MENSTRUAL CYCLE PHASES

Did you know there are four parts to your menstrual cycle?

It is not just once a month that we may feel a little different. Being a woman not only means we menstruate each month, but we are also on a rotating calendar of hormonal changes. These different parts to our cycle, however, can often be maintained by our diet.

Menstrual Phase

This is the phase we think of when we hear the words period or time of the month. Try and relax your body, it is already going through a lot. If you are used to exercising in your routine, do not push yourself if you do not fancy it, and maybe opt for a slow walk instead. Walking tends to help me with any period pain, but it is not for everyone. Extra iron during this time may be needed due to the loss of blood. Red meat, beans, tuna, and tofu are just a few options that include iron, or if you do struggle, your doctor will be able to provide you with medication.

Follicular Phase

Following our period, we are in the follicular phase for usually around a week. This is when two different hormones are released, FSH and LH which stimulate the growth and release of eggs in our ovaries.

During this time, we may have a boost of energy due to the extra production of oestrogen in our bodies, but this may also cause a decrease in appetite. Eating foods rich in fibre and phytoestrogen such as flax seeds, pomegranate, and dried mango may be beneficial in this stage.

### Ovulatory Phase

In this stage, our eggs are all ready to be fertilised. The ovary releases an egg, which goes along the fallopian tube and into the womb. You may experience some cramping due to ovulation, and a decrease in appetite as well as your mood. For this stage, remain eating a well-balanced diet rich in fibre, but you may also want to up your intake of magnesium and zinc, in which you can get a substantial amount from beans, nuts, and leafy greens. Ovulation only lasts around 3 days so if you are experiencing any pain, this should not last long.

### Luteal Phase

This phase unfortunately means potential bloating, spots, and fatigue, and you may also experience some anxiety. Cramping typically occurs during the menstrual stage, but some may experience a bit of pain in this stage too. The lining of the womb starts to thicken, in preparation for a possible pregnancy if an egg was fertilised. This is when you are most likely to experience a few cravings. Personally, the week before my period is due I have a chocolate craving when normally my go-to treat would be crisps, so this for me is my biggest giveaway that my period is due. You may also have an appetite increase which is perfectly normal during this time. I, for one, cannot stop eating the week before my period. Now is the time to eat whatever you fancy but in moderation of course.

So, let me break it down. What exactly is happening during your cycle?

Days 1-5 (Menstrual Phase)
During this time, you will have your period and bleed.

Days 6-14 (Follicular Phase)
The days after your period are when your body starts to build its endometrial lining again, which will keep building up until your next period.

Day 14 (Ovulatory Phase)
Ovulation is typically around halfway through your cycle. This is based on a 28-day cycle and is when an egg is released.

Days 15-28 (Luteal Phase)

The days after you ovulate are when your body is preparing for your next period and the endometrial lining continues to thicken.

## PERIODS

This is something you will all experience at some point in your teenage years and quite frankly, it can be rubbish, I am not going to lie to you.

I personally have struggled with my periods for a while now, from fainting on holiday, to an ambulance turning up at work. Fun times! I started my period when I was 15. I was always quite thin, and my body developed a lot later than most of my friends, but this is nothing to be embarrassed about. I am actually quite thankful, as some of my friends started their periods at 10 years old, so at least I had a few extra years.

Question time.

If you have just started your period, or you are at the age where it is soon to start, you may have a few questions. If you are anything like I was, you may be too shy to ask anyone, so I hope this helps.

"Why do we get periods?"

Your body is incredible and so clever. Every month your body goes through a cycle called the menstrual cycle, which on average is about 28 days, but this varies from person to person. My cycle is around 23 days, just as an example. The cycle is worked out by counting from the first day of your period, up until the day before your next period. It is also normal for this to change each month by a few days so do not panic.

"Will it be painful?"
Again, different with everyone, but I highly doubt your first few periods will be painful. You may never experience much pain; a lot of my friends do not really get any pain at all, and they do not feel any different to any other day. Personally, mine got worse over the years. If you ever experience huge amounts of pain I would recommend booking an appointment with your doctor. I was always rather shy when it came to talking about my periods until I was reassured it is normal, and other people experience the same as me.

Period cramps are unfortunately something you may experience due to your uterus contracting and pushing the unneeded endometrial lining out of your body through your vagina when an egg is not fertilised.

Some months may be worse than others pain-wise, due to the fluctuation of hormones, but there are a few things you could do to make it a little more bearable.

Regular exercise is top of the list, and although this is not enjoyable for everyone, and I of all people cannot stand exercise, it can help increase your blood flow which will ease the cramping. You do not have to overdo it, just a simple walk will do.

Remaining hydrated can help reduce water retention and bloating. Girls will typically feel bloated during their period, so keeping up with your water intake can also help reduce cramping. It may seem strange to drink a lot of water when feeling bloated but trust me, it works.

Ensuring you increase your intake of healthy foods and eating a balanced diet with plenty of fruit and vegetables, will also help. If you can also avoid caffeine this will work to your advantage, as caffeine naturally dehydrates you and may contribute to bloating.

Get plenty of rest and let your body relax, to help reduce cramps. Applying heat is an effective way to get your muscles to relax, as tensing can often cause cramps. Hot water bottles or a nice warm bath would be perfect, just make sure when using hot water bottles that you have adult supervision.

Sleep. Ensuring you also have enough sleep each night will benefit you, as you need around eight hours of sleep per night, especially on your period, to help you feel refreshed each day.

If these home remedies do not work for you, a trip to the chemist for some over-the-counter pain relief medication may be necessary or a visit to the doctors.

"What should it look like?"

I was not going to add this in, but I then remembered there were a few times I have looked at the toilet paper or in my underwear and worried because of what it looked like. The colour of the blood will be different for everyone depending on how heavy you are, but mine tends to be brown or dark red at the start and end, then bright red in the middle. This is normal as brown or dark red is just old blood, and bright red is fresh.

If you experience any orange or grey blood, this calls for professional advice as this may be a sign of a bacterial infection. Watch out for itching, burning, and bad smells too. You may also experience a few clots, and these can vary in size but are also completely normal for those suffering from heavy periods.

"What happens at night?"
Your period flow naturally slows as you are lying down, but I would suggest if you do use tampons, to also use a pad for extra protection at night, as it will be left longer than during the day, and waking up with blood in your bed is never fun, trust me. You may also experience a rush of blood when you first stand up in the morning, due to gravity. If you just use pads, I would suggest using night time ones as these are thicker and have wings

for added protection as you move in your sleep.

I tend to stay up late on the days my period is heavy and set an early alarm so that my chances of leaking are as slim as possible. Please also note that you should only have a tampon in for a maximum of 8 hours, so you may want to switch to using pads at night instead, if you would like a long sleep.

"Will my period blood clot?"
Yes, it may do, and this is rather common unless they are large clots. Clots larger than a 10 pence piece are worth getting checked out, but anything smaller should not be anything to worry about. The first time I had a few clots, I noticed them on the toilet paper but also in the toilet and it worried me, but I can

assure you as long as they are not too large, this is normal and nothing to be worried about. If you do have any concerns though, do not hesitate to go and see your doctor just to be sure.

"How long will it last?"
It will probably feel like it is lasting forever, but it should only last 2-5 days. If you are unlucky it could last as long as 10 days. My first few periods were under 5 days but as I got older they seemed to get heavier and more painful, as well as last longer, so it entirely depends on your own body and hormones.

"When should I expect my next period?"
I remember being at school and dreading my period starting. It seemed to always happen first thing in the morning, and I was normally

a few days late. We are all different but there are apps available for your phone where you fill in when you start your period, and then again when it ends, and after a few months of logging your periods it will give you a rough idea of when your next one is likely to be, unless yours are completely irregular which unfortunately can be the case. I have had the app for a while now and it is pretty much spot on.

I will say though, once you have started your period, just make sure you always carry sanitary pads or tampons with you. They do not take up much room in your bag, and it definitely will be a lifesaver if you do ever come on unexpectedly.

"Will I have my period forever?"

Thankfully not, but most women will have their period until they go through menopause at around the age of 50. This is when your body goes through more hormonal changes and your ovaries stop producing eggs, meaning you are no longer able to have children. Do not panic about these changes yet though, as you have plenty of years ahead of you before then.

"How much is heavy bleeding?"

Heavy bleeding for one woman may be normal for another, so it is difficult to define exactly, as a period varies from woman to woman. Online it says the average amount of blood to lose during your period is less than 16 teaspoons (80ml), with the majority being around 6 to 8 teaspoons. Losing more than

80ml of blood during your period is considered heavy bleeding. Personally, I would say a good indication would be if you have to change your sanitary products every hour or two, if you bleed through your clothes, are passing large blood clots, or if you have to double up on products, for example using pads as well as tampons.

Heavy periods are rather common but can affect your daily life, and if you are concerned, talk to your GP who may be able to help.

In nearly half of all women with heavy periods, there is no underlying reason and it is just pure bad luck, but there are several conditions of the womb and ovaries that can be the cause so it is always best to check.

"Is my period normal?"

Most of you reading this will not need to worry, as you potentially have not even started your period yet, or you have only recently started, but for the first few years after starting your period, unfortunately irregular is categorised as normal, so within this time it is common to miss a period. This is also common for those who do a lot of strenuous exercise, those on strict diets, or even those feeling anxious or stressed, as your body is very sensitive to change.

Things to look out for:

- Your period lasts longer than 7 days
- Large clots
- Severe pain
- Bleeding in between periods
- Sudden changes with your cycle

- Missing a period for 6 months or more
- Soaking through a pad or tampon hourly

"What do I need?"

I was not prepared for my first period. Hopefully your parent will have sanitary products ready for you, but maybe have a conversation with them, just to check. If you need to buy them yourself, I recommend getting some light tampons or pads, whichever you feel you would be more comfortable using, as you should not bleed too much on your first period.

When it comes to buying yourself some pads or tampons, it can be a little intimidating with the large selection, but try not to worry as once you know your body and your cycle, you will know what to buy. After a few periods, you will start to notice how heavy your flow is, but to start with, I would recommend just getting a variety and perhaps start using the lower absorbency ones first.

Pads are fine, and if you feel more comfortable using thicker ones, then that is completely your decision, but when it comes to tampons, if you use larger ones and your flow is not very heavy, they can then cause irritation and be painful to remove. With tampons, you will know if you have chosen the correct absorbency, as your tampon will slide out easily without any pain, after the recommended time to take it out. If the tampon is sore to remove and seems dry, then you will know to change to using ones with a lower absorbency rating. This is the same for if you end up having any leakage, or have to remove your tampon more often than you should, you will know to go up a size. It can take time to find out what works best for you, but to avoid any upset or pain, I would start small and go from there. As a guide, if you need to change your tampon more often than every 4 hours, you should be using a higher absorbency rating.

I suggest getting some painkillers such as ibuprofen or paracetamol if you do end up experiencing any pain. There are also some great painkillers aimed at period cramps that you can get over the counter.

Once you have had a few periods and feel more comfortable, there are now other options such as the menstrual cup.

My Menstrual cup story

I got to a point where I was changing super plus tampons nearly every hour on my heavy days. This is not practical with any full-time job and is just inconvenient. The menstrual cup is environmentally friendly and lasts for years, which if you are a tampon or pad user, you will not only save a lot of money each year, but also the disposal during your lifetime, of around 11,000 tampons and pads, which is life-changing for both yourself, and the environment. I was fortunate when trying the cup for the first time that I had very detailed messages from a friend with her tips and tricks when it comes to inserting and removing the cup.

Day one of my period came and it was time to attempt to insert it. I am going to be honest, I was rather excited to give it a go after hearing stories from friends about how life-changing their experiences were. I folded the cup in half, put it in, and felt it open up inside which was rather strange. You may also hear a puff of air as it opens up, but this just confirms insertion was successful. It was a little tricky I must admit, and there is an element of shoving to get it inside, but overall it was not painful. It felt a little strange as obviously, it was all new to me, but give it a little time and you will not even notice it is in there, just the same as when using tampons. I had read and heard a few horror stories when it came to removing the cup so this was my worry.

When the time came for me to remove it, and given I had numerous tips from my friend when it came to removal, I felt ready to tackle the situation. However, when it came to it, I felt as if either the cup or my insides were going to break. I just could not grab it and felt as if every time I pulled it to try and pinch the cup and release the suction, it would just slide back up.

Finally, I got it and just kept pulling until it was out, which actually hurt. I was then given an incredible tip by a friend after mentioning to her that I struggled with removal, and she advised me to push my muscles as if I am going for a wee, and to then pull the cup at the same time until only the top rim was still inside, then using a finger to bring the rest out. I have realised after doing a little research though, that the cup can be inserted and removed using various techniques, so it is all about just finding what works for you. I did notice I was a little sore for a few days after my period, but that was probably because it was all new to me.

My first period using the menstrual cup was an overall positive experience. No leaking and I could leave it in for far longer than a tampon. Sadly since then, after numerous messy situations, I decided to go back to using tampons which I feel far more comfortable with, but as I have said before, it is all a personal preference. I felt the need to share as I know it has been incredible for numerous people, just unfortunately not me.

"Do periods smell?"
It is not bad, but menstruation does produce a slight smell which if you wear pads, might be more noticeable. Just remember to change

your pad regularly and this should not be a concern. If you are self-conscious about it, perhaps give tampons a try, as this will reduce the smell due to it collecting the blood inside the body.

"Should I use Pads or Tampons?"
This is completely up to you and your personal preference. Pads are a form of absorbency that you stick inside your underwear to absorb your flow once it leaves your body, whereas tampons are inserted into your vagina to absorb your flow before it leaves your body. Whether you choose to use pads or tampons is entirely up to you.

I use tampons but will use pads as well, on heavy days for extra protection. It feels safer having the blood inside me rather than in my underwear, plus the possibility of a pad moving and the blood ending up elsewhere worries me, but as long as you feel comfortable, the decision is yours. Most girls will start using pads first, but it is fine if you want to go straight into using tampons, I did. Perhaps chat to someone close to you and find out their opinions if you are struggling to decide. Tampons, however, do mean that you can continue all your usual daily activities including swimming without any worry, wear any outfit, including a bikini due to the invisibility.

"Do Tampons hurt?"

No, they should not hurt. If you put it in correctly, and are using the right size to suit your body and absorbency, then you should not even feel it. If it is uncomfortable and feels like it is not in properly, no worries, just take it out and insert a new one, this happens. I use tampons now without an applicator, but I would recommend using ones with an applicator to start with, so that insertion is easier and more comfortable.

"When do I change my tampon?"
So, because all our bodies are different, this is not a question I can answer that will be the same for everyone. You unfortunately will not know when the tampon is ready to come out as it is not anything we can feel, as far as I am aware, but after a little while, you will be able to work out how long to leave it in for roughly. Each day of your period will also be different, as the heaviness of your flow will change each day, but do not worry, this is something you will get used to.

When I first started my period, I had quite a few accidents, and this can be rather embarrassing, so I would suggest whilst you get used to wearing tampons and working out the time in between changing them, I would keep a liner or pad in your underwear as protection. Even at my age now, I have accidents so do not worry if it happens to you, as this again is normal. For me, in the final days of my period I can leave my tampon in for roughly 4 hours, but during the first few days when I am much heavier, I am often changing my tampon every hour. This however, is not normal, and if you are experiencing the same as me, I would suggest seeking a doctor's opinion as there may be an underlying issue.

Just a little tip. I would suggest either changing your tampon at times you can remember, or setting alarms on your phone, as this will help reduce the possibility of leaking. Our days can become busy, and if you are dosed up on painkillers or are not experiencing any pain, it is easy to forget.

"Can I go to the toilet whilst using a tampon?" This is a question I am sure most girls have googled. I, for one, have, and the answer is yes, you can, but you may prefer not to. It entirely depends on how often you change your tampon and whether you need the toilet in between. I have to change mine regularly, so I would go the same time as putting a new tampon in, but for those who can last quite a few hours without needing to change it, do not waste a tampon just for the sake of it, as it is perfectly fine to go to the toilet with it still in.

"How to avoid tampon leaks?"

Tampons may ensure certain outfits and activities are possible, but there is always that worry deep down of leaking. Tampons can of course leak, but this will mainly be if they are left for too long. Tampons, unlike pads, are hidden, so unless you take the tampon out, you will not be able to tell how full it is. Do not panic though, it is all trial and error, and it may take a little while to get into a routine. Perhaps you need to choose a higher absorbency though if your tampon needs changing too often. Consider that the heaviness of your period will also change daily, so you may need to change your tampon more regularly for the first few days. Stock up on a few different absorbency options so that you are prepared for the daily changes when on your period.

"How do I insert a tampon?"
This can be a little intimidating especially if it is your first time, but I can assure you it really is rather simple, you just have to make sure you are comfortable and relaxed. Finding a comfortable position will help with insertion. I find standing with my knees bent in a sort of squatting position is the best way, but this is just my personal preference. Once in a comfortable position, hold the tampon applicator using your thumb and index finger, and insert gently into your vagina, ensuring a couple of centimetres are inside. Then with your middle finger, push the inner tube until it is fully inside the outer tube, as this then

slides the tampon inside. You should not be able to feel the tampon unless you were to put your fingers inside, so if you can feel it, you know it is not in far enough. Inside the packaging, you should find a step-by-step guide with images if you get stuck. Just relax, you will be a professional in no time.

"How do I remove a tampon?"
Tampons are designed to be easily removed. They have a piece of string attached to them that goes through the centre of the tampon, ensuring the string does not come off and leave the tampon behind. When you are ready to remove your tampon, simply pull on the string and it should slide straight out with ease. This should then be wrapped and put in a sanitary bin, as tampons should not be

flushed down the toilet, however, a lot of people do flush them.

"Can a tampon get lost?"
You can relax as the short answer is no. Your tampon will not get lost inside you because of how your body is built. The end of your vagina is closed off by your cervix which only has a tiny opening. A tampon cannot pass from the vagina through the cervix to your uterus, so there is nowhere for your tampon to go. There may be times where you cannot find the string due to this folding inside your vagina, but it is important not to panic, as like I have said above, it cannot go anywhere, so just relax, and using your fingers, gently feel for it, and pull it out. If you have given it a good shot and still cannot get it out, a trip to the doctors is recommended as leaving a tampon in for too

long can cause infection. They see this all the time so there is no need to find this embarrassing, and ensuring your tampon is removed will prevent any sort of infection. Most GP surgeries will let you see a female doctor if you prefer.

Cravings/Emotions

I have not ever really thought about cravings, although chocolate is top of the list the week before my period and I do have an increase in appetite. This then changes drastically when I am on my period and I pretty much have to force myself to eat due to the pain I am in most months. When it comes to emotions though, I can be honest and say I am extremely emotional the few days before my period and can switch drastically between any emotion, from crying to feeling angry, and this is perfectly normal for many. During my period, I would say I can be a tad short in conversation, but find if I explain myself, most will understand, as hormones can do insane things to your body and mental state.

Anaemia

Occasionally, if you have heavy periods, it can cause anaemia which unfortunately is a serious health condition. Essentially it is an iron deficiency and it occurs when a person does not have enough red blood cells, or their haemoglobin levels are low. Haemoglobin is vital, it is an iron-rich protein in your red blood cells that carries oxygen to your body's organs and tissues via the blood.

Anaemia can result in weakness and fatigue and some may even pass out or faint in severe cases, of which I am one. Some may suffer from shortness of breath, often creating a challenge when it comes to fitness. Anaemia can be genetic but women are at a higher risk of iron deficiency due to blood loss during menstruation.

Medication can be prescribed for severe cases, but often changing your diet and including iron-rich foods can do wonders. Try also adding Vitamin C into your daily diet when eating foods rich in iron, as this can help support the absorption of iron into your body.

## TOXIC SHOCK SYNDROME (TSS)

This is very rare, but it is a life-threatening condition caused by toxins due to bacteria entering the body. This can affect anyone at any age but is mostly seen in young women and is associated with tampons. However rare this condition is, it is important to be aware of it so that you can take action if needed and it can be diagnosed early and treated successfully. The link between TSS and tampons is due to the absorbency, which is why I strongly advise that when using tampons, you always use the lowest absorbency rating possible to suit your menstrual flow. This, however scary it sounds, should not be a reason to stop using tampons as there is no evidence to say the material used to make tampons increases or leads to toxins being produced to cause TSS.

Symptoms of TSS:

- High temperature
- Low blood pressure
- Vomiting
- Diarrhoea
- Confusion
- Sore throat
- Fainting or feeling faint
- Muscle pain
- Irritated skin
- Dizziness

You may only experience a couple of these symptoms, but unfortunately, anyone at any age can get TSS so it is highly advised to be seen by a professional if you do experience any symptoms. TSS is not always caused by tampons, it is also commonly caused by burns and insect bites, and even if you have had TSS once, this does not mean you are immune to getting it again. If you have had TSS already, it is advised that you see a doctor before using tampons again.

If diagnosed early, TSS treatment can be given, and there is a high chance of a full recovery. The total count of fatal cases is extremely low, just to put your mind at ease. Change your tampon regularly, and ensure that even when sleeping, you do not leave it in for longer than 8 hours. Always use the lowest absorbency rating to suit your menstrual flow, and make sure you remove the tampon before putting a new one in. An embarrassing story for you, that relates to this, is that I forgot once, and put another tampon in, which then got stuck. I managed after about 4 hours to get this out, although I decided after some persuading from a friend that I should get it checked to make sure, and it turns out I had another full tampon inside me. I still, to this day, have no idea how long that was in there for, so make sure you only use a tampon when needed, and never as protection for when you are due on, to avoid situations like mine.

## IRREGULAR PERIODS

Countless things can cause irregular periods. If you have recently started your period, then I would not worry too much if they are irregular as it can take a while for your body to fully adjust, but for those that have had their periods for years and they are still struggling with regularity, then there are a few factors to take into consideration.

Stress is most likely the number one cause of any changes in the regularity of your periods. You may find your periods were regular and like clockwork, then you have important exams coming up or something happening in your life that has caused your emotions to spike, and your periods change. This is normal as your body can be massively affected by your emotions, and while stress should be taken seriously, your periods should go back to normal once your emotions settle down. If you are feeling it has changed too drastically though, do not hesitate to contact your doctor to discuss options.

Diet and exercise can also play a huge part when it comes to irregular periods. I find that when I include exercise into my routine, and am eating a healthier balanced diet overall, that my regularity and pain are noticeably better. You may notice that changes in your bowel movements coincide with your period pattern, and find that a change of diet or exercise in your routine can also affect you.

There are many reasons why your periods may be irregular. It could be a medical condition, an infection, a hormonal imbalance, or a wide range of other factors, which is why it is best, before jumping to any conclusions, to consult a professional if you do have any worries, as they are there to help.

## MY PERIOD STORY

I can remember my first period as if it were yesterday. I was going to the New Forest with my family, and a few minutes before we were about to leave IT HAPPENED. Talk about bad timing. I went to talk to my mum which at the time I was very shy about, but at the end of the day, she is my mum. I told her, and she said she knew this would happen soon so had kept a few things stored away in preparation. Bless her, she explained it all to me and said it was my choice what I wanted to use, but without a doubt, I went straight to using tampons, and I have not looked back since. They are so easy to use, although they may look a little scary at first, but trust me, it feels a lot better than having a thick pad in your pants just getting in the way. I could continue with all my activities like normal, which for me was great as my mum was a swimming instructor at the time, and we used to go swimming often, so for me using tampons was the best option. I am honestly so glad I started using tampons right from the beginning as I know a few of my friends are still anxious now to use them, having always used pads since day one.

The first year I was lucky and it really did not affect my life in the slightest, but this then changed. The older I got, the worse it became.

On the first and second day of my period pretty much every month, I would feel rather sick and weak, and occasionally I would faint too. With age, my pain became worse, and the heaviness of it too, so after months of fainting and being sick, I finally got the courage to see a doctor. I always had a fear of doctors, I am not sure why, as they really are all so lovely and I had not had any bad experiences. It was just a little phobia of mine, along with spiders.

I found it embarrassing to talk about periods at first, but it now seems to be a daily topic for me. I was given the contraceptive pill to try, which I took for 21 days and would then have a week's break. This worked and really helped me at first, but I then got some rather bad side effects such as migraines, so they switched me to another pill. After trying five different pills over the years, I stopped taking it completely to give my body a break and to see if I could manage without it. For a few months, I was fine, and then suddenly, my periods became really bad every month again. The office where I used to work even had to call an ambulance out once, as my blood pressure had dropped drastically, and I was in unbelievable amounts of pain to the point where I could not walk, I was shaking, and being physically sick. There was not anything they could give me or do about it so back to the doctors I went, which is when I was offered the coil in an attempt to level my hormones out. This caused me more discomfort than anything else, and even though my periods were lighter, I was also getting random pain and bleeding throughout the month too. Back to the doctors I went again, but this time they did a few ultrasound scans which alerted them that a few things were not quite right.

I was then booked in for an operation called a Laparoscopy, which is where a tiny camera goes inside you to have a look around. For me, they did not resolve anything by doing that and I was put back on the contraceptive pill, although this time it was the mini pill, which you take every single day, in the hope to stop your periods completely. This I took for around three years and although I still had a lot of pain, the severity of it decreased. It settled my periods a little but never stopped them as the doctor had hoped, so I came off the pill completely to give my body another break. At this point I had been on a contraceptive pill for around 10 years which is not advised without a proper break. I then pushed to see a gynaecologist, and after six months of appointments and scans, I was booked in for another laparoscopy to remove an ovarian cyst and was also diagnosed with endometriosis.

I have noticed my mental health is also massively affected by my periods. This is normal for anyone, due to the possible hormonal imbalance, but as I feel so unwell with mine I am working on ways to resolve these feelings. I have focused on my self-care recently, to ensure my mental health is more controlled. Coping mechanisms that work for me, such as meditation and journaling, are good ways to release my emotions, but it may take time to find what works for you. Make sure you give time for yourself, self-care is important and I for one do not do enough of it.

I really hope my story has helped those who suffer with their periods, and that you now realise you are not alone and that there are so many people out there wanting to help you.

Please do not push it aside, doctors are there for you and the sooner you get help, the sooner you can start feeling better.

Secret little tips-

Pad/Tampon cases

Cases can make your time of the month a little more discreet. You can buy these online and they come in pretty patterns so that no one will ever know if they look in your bag. You could also get a coin purse and fit them in there, as that is what I do as my current handbag does not have a zipped pocket.

Discreet toilet trips

Just a little something I do when out and about, is to hide my tampon up my sleeve or in my pocket so that I am not telling the whole office that I am on my period by taking my handbag with me to the toilet. Obviously, this is a little trickier in the summer, but the trick is to plan your outfits a little better that week and to maybe wear a long top covering your back pockets if you do not have long sleeves due to the weather for example.

Period first aid kit

Definitely one for those who are due to start or have just started recently and have not had enough time to get to know what their periods are like yet.

Create a little section in your bag or even get yourself a pretty new makeup bag and put the below things into it.

- Pads
- Tampons

- Paracetamol
- Spare underwear
- Wipes and tissues

This is then discrete but also super handy and means you will always be prepared.

## ENDOMETRIOSIS

For those that don't know, endometriosis is a chronic long-term condition that occurs when tissue similar to the lining of the womb grows elsewhere in the body such as on the ovaries.

Endometriosis takes an average of around eight years to be diagnosed, which is why it is so important for young girls to be aware of the signs, and to be aware of what is considered normal or not. Symptoms can vary from person to person, but the majority will experience severe period pains with heavy bleeding, vomiting, diarrhoea, pelvic and hip pain, as well as bloating. Endometriosis can sometimes also result in fertility issues.

My periods vary massively. Some months the pain is manageable with prescribed medication, and other months even the strongest dose my doctor can give me will not even touch the sides. Bad months for me happen far too regularly, but I have not worked out what the trigger is yet, as each month seems to differ so I never know what to expect until the day. I have found that certain things like exercise, for example, do help, so I try to exercise as often as I can without forcing myself, as you do also have to listen and be mindful of your body and what it needs.

This past year I had a few blood tests which brought up concerns with my doctor. I was diagnosed with anaemia and have been prescribed tablets to help. Iron deficiency anaemia is rather common in those with heavy periods, and in my case, endometriosis. A bad period, which I suppose my endometriosis can be partially blamed for, consists of bleeding through high absorbency tampons nearly every hour, being sick, fainting or feeling extremely weak resulting in the lack of ability to drive or even stand for too long, and an unmanageable level of pain.

However much I hate the fact I have endometriosis, I am slightly relieved having had a diagnosis as I have spent far too much of my life already in and out of doctors surgeries, hospitals and having scan appointments. However much this is not over, and it is really only the start of my journey, at least I can relax because I now know what is wrong and can focus on managing my symptoms.

I am hugely grateful for having found a fantastic consultant after struggling every month for many years. I was always just told I have bad periods. Mild pain and discomfort during your period as a teenager or an adult can be normal, however, if this pain affects your daily life, this needs to be looked into. Period pain should be manageable with over the counter painkillers such as paracetamol, but if it is not, you should be seen by a professional. Periods are nothing to be embarrassed about, and if you are suffering, please do not push this aside. Your health is important.

## Diagnosis

To enable a diagnosis to be made, a laparoscopic procedure needs to be done. This is a type of keyhole surgery where a thin tube with a camera is put through a small incision inside your belly button to look at your pelvic area. Small incisions may also need to be made further down in order to investigate properly. Endometriosis cannot be diagnosed without this surgery, but doctors and specialist consultants will be able to notice symptoms and signs by tests, an ultrasound scan and perhaps an MRI first.

## FEAR OF THE SMEAR

I completely understand that when it comes to having your first smear test, it can be nerve-racking. Cervical screening rates are at their lowest in decades, and whilst I understand it is completely your choice, I hope after reading this, you will put your health before embarrassment, and go for your cervical smear test when it is due.

Lying on a bed with your legs wide open having a nurse feel around inside can be rather embarrassing for some, especially if it is your first time, but those few moments of embarrassment can potentially save you from cervical cancer, and in theory, save your life.

Most of you reading this now will be too young, as you will not recieve your first letter to book your test until you reach the age of 24, but I want to mention the fact that it is ok. I had my first smear when I was 26, which was much later than recommended, but I, like others, was petrified of going. However nervous you are, I can assure you it is fine, and the nurse will make you feel as comfortable as she can. It is also over within a few minutes, and all that worry will be for nothing.

## VAGINAL DISCHARGE

This is something that, once you hit puberty, you may notice in your underwear. Vaginal discharge varies in appearance, and the time of the month affects it. Discharge is normally nothing to worry about and changes throughout the month are normal. It is mucus or fluid that keeps the vagina clean and helps prevent infections. Your vagina is self-cleaning, how cool is that?

What does vaginal discharge look like?
Discharge varies in texture and colour depending on your cycle. It is usually clear or white in colour and it can be jelly-like, thick or thin in texture. This can change to have a hint of brown or red when your period is due. The amount of discharge varies from person

to person, but you can use pantyliners that offer light protection, and these can be changed throughout the day for freshness if you fancy it, or feel the need. I personally do not suffer from discharge, but around the time of my period I may get a little, but it is not ever really anything to worry about or use a liner or pad for. You may notice certain times in the month you will experience discharge and the rest of the month is dry and this is also normal.

It may be a sign of infection if your discharge changes from what is normal for you, for example if the colour, smell, or texture changes. Here are a few things to look out for.

- Smells fishy
- Green or yellow in colour

- Frothy in texture
- With pelvic pain or bleeding when not on your period
- With sores or blisters

## BODY HAIR

Body hair is different for everyone, and the age you start getting it also varies from person to person. I was a late bloomer, and I do not think I started shaving until I was around 15 years old, around the same time I started my period. I may have been unlucky with my periods, but when it comes to body hair, I am extremely fortunate. I opted for shaving as it is pain-free unless you cut yourself, which can sting a lot, but it should not bleed for longer than a few minutes and is quick to heal.

Luckily for me, my hair takes a while to grow back, and I can often go around three weeks without the need to shave my legs or bikini area. My underarms I only need to shave once a week, but I do have some friends who need to shave daily so your hair growth rate will be unique to you.

There are many different methods of hair removal. Everyone is different and I would recommend trying a few options, to see which suits you best. I have stuck to using a razor, as it is pain-free, and as I mentioned above, my hair takes a while to grow back, so I do not feel a lot of effort or time goes into my hair removal routine. If you suffer from dark hair, or it grows back quickly then you may want to look at alternatives to shaving such as waxing, and if you have any facial hair I would recommend not using a razor for this.

## WEIGHT CHANGE

This is something not everyone will experience. I know of a few friends who can eat anything and everything and still struggle to maintain and gain weight, but then some put on weight no matter what they eat. We are all different.

I was always quite thin growing up. I would eat a normal balanced diet along with fast food like anybody else, but I always remained the same weight until I was about 18 years old, which I put down to hormonal changes. This is not me trying to boast, as I know a lot of people who put weight on no matter how healthy their diet is, but I am just trying to point out that everyone is different, and either of the above can be daily struggles for a lot of people. If you are struggling with either weight gain or loss, perhaps seeing a doctor would be advisory, especially if this could be detrimental to your health in the long run. If a healthy diet, combined with regular exercise is not benefiting you with your weight change, perhaps it could be an underlying health issue or a hormone imbalance. My iron levels being low caused me to lose weight quite drastically in a short space of time, and only when I was prescribed medication, did my weight go back to normal for me.

Body size and weight affects a lot of us daily, but what people do not realise is that it is not just those that are gaining weight that are struggling, it is also those that find it a challenge to put weight on. You never know what people are going through so just make sure you are considerate of others when mentioning weight change.

**BRAS**

As I am writing this I am trying to think of the age I was when I started wearing a bra. I honestly cannot remember, but what I do know, is that I was later than most of my friends. I was never bothered by the fact I developed later than most, as things like periods are not fun, and still to this day I struggle with them. I know from speaking with friends though, that starting your period or getting boobs can be a big thing to some, and a way of showing maturity. This I completely understand, but you should love your body the way it is, however hard that may be during certain stages of your life. Having larger boobs is also not everything. Trust me. You may regret wishing for large boobs when you get older, as things like sports bras make your body ache, regardless of the amount of exercise you have done. I wish I were one of those girls who could leave the house and be able to wear a bralette without the worry of it not being supportive enough. However, if I wear a baggy hoodie, I can get away with it, as the lack of support is not noticeable.

For those with larger boobs, finding that perfect bra that is flattering, pretty, but also supportive can be a challenge. I have found over the years that getting a bra fitting is the way forward, and if you choose a shop you love, the chances are that once you have been fitted, you will be able to find something to suit your style, as well as giving you the support you need.

Bra fittings are unfortunately something you may need to do on a regular basis though, depending on your body. As your weight fluctuates, which being a girl and having hormone levels constantly changing, is completely normal, you may find the way your bra fits also changes. Other things can contribute to changes in your bra size, such as hormones, diet, exercise regime, age, and pregnancy. I suppose we are in for a lifetime of new bras.

## SKIN

Another easily judged topic. Growing up I was fortunate enough not to suffer from spots or acne, so I cannot speak from my own experience, but again a lot of my friends and people I know have unfortunately suffered, and a fair few of them were also prescribed medication after trying a load of different products and not having any luck.

When it comes to skincare, most of us will turn to products, and will fall for the expensive posh-looking products too, thinking this will be the best outcome for our skin, when outer beauty actually comes from within. Yes, products are something to factor into your routine, but perhaps the below will be far more beneficial and will also save yours or your parent's bank account too.

What can help?

Healthy Diet

Eating a diet enriched with plenty of fruit and vegetables, protein, and healthy fats such as avocados, salmon, and eggs, will help keep your skin looking young and hydrated, as well as also helping to reduce inflammation. Your younger years are the prime time to focus on maintaining that healthy diet. Some people find that reducing gluten or dairy in their diet helps improve their skin, but it may be worth talking to a nutritionist before making any drastic changes.

Water

Remaining hydrated is key, and probably the most important step to take when looking after your skin (and your overall health of course). Your cells are around 60% water, so staying hydrated will help when it comes to keeping your cells healthy, as well as keeping the elasticity of the skin to help against premature ageing.

Sugar

Limiting, or at least lowering your sugar intake. Too much sugar in your body leads to the loss of collagen and elastin, which are both vital for youthful, healthy skin. If you are a fizzy drink lover, this is the first recommended place to start. Finding that alternative replacement beverage without the high sugar count will do the world of good.

This does not mean you have to cut out sugar in your diet, but everything in moderation is key.

Vitamins

Eating foods such as broccoli and citrus fruits that are high in Vitamin C, can help your collagen levels, which helps the signs of UVB induced photoaging. This is premature skin ageing caused by overexposure to the sun's rays.

Stress

Everyday stress can play a huge part in the quality of your skin. Try and focus on your self-care to ensure your skin does not suffer because of how you feel.

## Skin Imperfections

Stretch marks are sadly something we may struggle to love, and can often feel the need to edit images or add filters to hide them. As mentioned previously, learning to love yourself and your body for how it is will have such an impact on your life and emotions. If you are unhappy with your body, then by all means change it, but stretch marks are often tricky to get rid of, and it is far better to work on embracing it, rather than letting it affect your mentality.

In a way, these are scars, and you may not think they are pretty, but accepting them and realising they are a part of beautiful you, means they are beautiful too. When I first noticed I developed stretch marks, I instantly thought it must mean I am overweight, but this is not the case as even the skinniest of people get them. Stretch marks are nothing to be ashamed of.

Cellulite and uneven skin tones are other things girls seem to stress about and get upset over. Perfect does not exist, and the sooner you realise this, the better, as every single person in this world has body hang-ups, but this does not mean to say you are not beautiful, because you are, you just need to believe it.

Skin imperfections show a journey that is your life, and without them, you would not be you. They come with weight, growth and becoming an adult. It takes time for acceptance, and years of learning to love yourself, but you will get there I promise.

# *Confidence*

"EVERY ADVENTURE REQUIRES A FIRST STEP" -*Alice In Wonderland*

## LOVE YOUR BODY

Body confidence comes from within. Our bodies are unique, and it is just a case of realising that and loving your own. When scrolling through social media platforms, I look at photos wishing I had that figure, when actually, the majority of images online have been edited to be unrealistic. Any cellulite and stretch marks are edited out to give that flawless look, and unfortunately, this is how body confidence drops, and the wrong image is portrayed to young girls.

It is difficult being a woman I must admit. I feel there is a certain way we need to look to prevent us from getting hurtful comments. We are all different, and it is about time society realised this. It is always "she is too thin, too curvy, too fat, too tall, too short". Why can we not be loving towards each other? There should not be any expectations or judgements on how you look at all, and there is no perfect figure, as everyone is beautiful and should be loved for who they are, not for their body.

I hear and see this all the time about girls detoxing and dieting before their beach holiday, but let me reassure you, nobody needs an intense diet or detox beforehand. You should never feel the need to change, unless advised by a doctor due to health reasons, of course.

I have, however, a few tips that may help when it comes to feeling more confident on your summer holiday, as I know it can be a challenge for a lot of us.

### Waterproof mascara

I know it is advised not to wear makeup when you are in the sun as it is not any good for your skin at all, so if you feel comfortable without any on then that is great, but if you are anything like me, then you may feel the need for a little something. Just a tad of mascara makes me feel ten times better, but do not forget to buy a waterproof one, or you will end up resembling a panda after a dip in the pool or sea.

### The right swimwear for you

Now you may not be too fussed about swimwear and may be confident wearing anything, but for some, wearing a bikini or swimsuit can make you feel self-conscious. I would suggest finding one that compliments your figure and how you feel wearing it. If you do not like your tummy, for example, or you bloat easily, as we all love to eat more than usual on holiday, then there are plenty of options out there to cover you more. I tend to shop online, order a large selection in various sizes, and then send any back I am not keen on. If you rush this and end up having to panic buy, or need to take swimwear you do not feel comfortable in, this could potentially affect you negatively when the time comes to wearing it.

Get a tan

Fortunately for me, I only need a few hours or so in the sun to get a base tan, but for those of you that struggle to tan or perhaps do not tan at all, you may want to think about getting hold of some fake tan before you go away. I can guarantee you that once you have a tan, it will drastically boost your confidence. Be careful not to burn, and please ensure you use sunscreen to tan safely.

### Choosing your food wisely

Just before you panic, I am not saying you have to eat healthily, as, after all, you are on holiday, but when you are in swimwear daily, the last thing you want is to feel bloated. The heat, in my opinion, really does help when it comes to avoiding stodgy foods like chips and pasta, although I do eat plenty of ice cream, sorbet and crisps on holiday, so I guess that makes up for it. But, if you want your tummy to feel fabulous whilst on holiday, take my advice and have some lighter meals instead.

Stop comparing yourself

Finally, stop comparing yourself to others. You should never compare yourself to anyone else as you are you, just like the cover of my book says, but I know how hard it is not to, and I am still personally working on this myself. We have all been lying there on that sunbed looking at the person next to us, wishing we had those legs, those arms, or abs, but in reality, they will be doing the same thing to someone else, or even you. We all want what we do not have. Not a single person in this entire world loves every inch of their body, not even models. Start focusing on the things you love about yourself instead of putting yourself down.

Anyway, for those of you like me who feel the excitement after booking a holiday but then the complete panic of trying to get that beach body in time, all I can say is do not panic, as we all have a beach body, we just need to learn to love it.

We all seem to think that if we change our body, we will gain self-confidence. We feel if we look better, we will feel better. For me, changing my appearance makes me feel better, whether it is losing weight, toning or changing my hair, but let me tell you, it never lasts longer than a few days and is not a long-term fix. I will admit, though, that walking out of a hair salon after a cut and blow-dry does make me feel on top of the world, but after a few days I am back to being me. If anything, I would end up thinking of more things I want to change about myself, which understandably would end in my self-confidence decreasing. Once you can be happy with your appearance and accept who you are, you can improve your confidence around it, I promise. Try and focus on performance goals instead, and I can assure you your confidence will increase naturally as a result.

Do not get me wrong, there are things I still want to change about my body, like anyone, but I am also learning to love myself and see the positive in every aspect of myself, which I hope after reading this, you will too.

We are all different, and that is what makes us all unique.

When it comes to clothing and body shape, it is all about learning what suits you, as well as what you are comfortable in. There is no point wearing an outfit you look incredible in if your feelings do not match. Body confidence is not something that happens overnight. It is something to work on in your own time, to learn to feel how you should, no matter the size and shape of your body. We all have different body shapes, and once you know how to accentuate the right curves, finding that look to make you feel fabulous and confident will become far easier.

I once shared a photo online that included an unseen, unedited photo of me from the year before in slightly revealing clothing. It is a photo I would never have dreamt of posting before, so why, because there was an "after" photo, was it then acceptable in my mind to post it? We should not feel this way about our bodies. When I posted this photo, I was not even able to say one nice thing about myself in the "before" photo, and would just pick out the parts I disliked. This, unfortunately, is normal for a lot of people, especially girls.

Body confidence, I will be honest, has always been a slight issue for me, and those that know me personally will probably find it hard to pick a time where I have worn tight or revealing clothing, as I am always in baggy jumpers and hoodies and this is why. I had noticed this was becoming a larger issue in my life, and am still in the process of learning to love my body, as these things take time.

Learning to love and accept your body can be a huge thing to overcome for many of us. Looking in the mirror and pinching parts you want to disappear is common, but this is not how anyone should be thinking about their body. I have noted a few steps below that have helped me massively that I want to share.

Instagram cut

Things like social media can have such an influence on the way we look. I decided to cut down on those that I follow online to change my thought process when scrolling through. I now follow friends, and a small handful of other accounts, meaning any posts of influencers showing off their incredibly toned thin bodies, are kept to a minimum, as well as anything negative in general. I really cannot recommend this enough. There are far too many accounts that you may think are great, but they are only doing more harm in the long run. Perhaps they are portraying that perfect life, or they are showing themselves after a 30-day workout challenge, both of which are having a negative impact on your life without you perhaps even realising it at the time.

Positive healthy goals

If you are struggling to maintain a healthy lifestyle and perhaps are an all or nothing person when it comes to food and exercise like I am, maybe try and make a little plan with some basic small guidelines and tips for the week. If food is an issue, I find preparing meals works for me to stay on track and not get too distracted. Often the weeks where I eat everything in sight is due to laziness, and perhaps my mental health state, meaning I resort to what is called comfort eating. Having meals prepped and ready to reheat in the microwave in a few minutes helps eliminate the lazy option to just grab something quick, easy, and most likely unhealthy.

Uplifting notes

This is a recent learning of mine, but something that has helped when it comes to my self-esteem. Writing positive notes about yourself and sticking them on your bathroom mirror and your fridge, whether this is about your general life, ability, or body, and reading them out loud to yourself daily, can have such a positive impact on how you feel. I have a few body positive notes on my bathroom mirror that I read whilst brushing my teeth, and however much I do not believe them when I say them, over time, I can see it making a massive difference to how I talk and think about myself, and it will eventually become a habit.

Have you ever noticed that by changing something in your life, perhaps making your bed in the morning daily for a while, that you then go on to doing this automatically? If you do something every day, after just a short space of time, you will have formed a habit, which in theory is something you do without even thinking, and this will be the same for beliefs about yourself.

## INFLUENCE OF SOCIAL MEDIA

Social media nowadays has such an impact on a young girl's life, and no one seems to be themselves anymore as they are always trying to be someone else, whether it is with how they look or how they act. When I was a teenager, apps like Instagram did not exist. It does make me sad when I think back on how things used to be when I was growing up, compared to how they are now, and I honestly feel sorry for the younger generation. I was enjoying life with family and friends, not having to care about impressing my online followers. Yes, I had a phone, but I had limited calls and texts and a game called snake, which I am sure most have not even heard of now.

When I grew up there was no social media to worry about, and not everything was dependent on whether your outfit was on-trend, or how many followers and likes you had. I would be out on my bike meeting friends, as I could not really talk to them any other way as we did not have things like WhatsApp or Snapchat and had to be careful with how much credit we used, as each text cost money. I struggle to understand how the innovation of technology was meant to connect people, but ironically it has made many anti-social instead.

I have also noticed how young girls seem to look up to public figures and feel the need to look the same. Wearing dresses that are far too short, posting photos of themselves in bikinis, having a full face of makeup, and to top it off, they all have dark and fake looking eyebrows. It is all attention-seeking, but not in a good way, and to be honest, at the end of the day wearing that much makeup at such a young age is only going to result in bad skin and a face full of spots. I would highly recommend purchasing a good cleanser and night cream instead. You will thank me later.

I could go on for longer, listing all the changes between the adolescents of today and a decade before, but like most things in life, you have to take the good with the bad, and unless you go and live off the grid somewhere very far away with no signal, there is no escaping technology and the pressures of social media.

You can, however, change the way you see things and stop allowing it all to influence your life, and as a result, you might find yourself to be happier and possibly saner by just being yourself and not having a care in the world about people who have very little or no relevance in your day to day life.

So, here is a challenge, and believe me, I would not ask you to do anything that I would not do myself. Leave your phone for an hour or more each day this next week, and in that time, just step outside to breathe in the fresh air, take your dog for a walk, or sit and read a book. Once you have completed this for a week, write down three things in a notebook about how you felt after doing this.

## FEELING SHY

Right from day one, I have struggled with my confidence. I think the way I was brought up made a huge difference. My family is quite reserved and not one for inviting friends over all the time, so I never really had a lot of people around me, whereas a lot of my friends, their houses would be full of people daily, and for them, that was normal. I think, because I was not used to having large gatherings, I was never an outgoing or loud person growing up. In senior school, I would stick to my small group of friends, my normal daily routine (home, dinner, television, bath and bed), and I only ever saw friends after school on a Friday evening, or weekends. This is not me criticising the way I was brought up at all, I actually really enjoyed going home to a tidy and quiet house with dinner ready on the table, and a bath run for me (amazing, right!). Then I got to relax and watch television, and message my friends for a bit on MSN (before things like Snapchat and WhatsApp existed), and then it was time for bed so that I was refreshed to start all over again the following day.

From the age of 11, my mum decided I was a little too quiet I think (boy did she regret this) and signed me up to go to Guides so that I could make friends outside of school that had the same interests as me. I had been to Rainbows and Brownies, but most children are fairly confident at that age and happy to play with anyone. I honestly cannot thank my mum enough for persuading me to go that very first time as I have made friends for life.

Anyways, I have gone a little off track. What I am trying to say, is that things like joining Guides were challenging for me as I was always so shy when it came to meeting new people, but now, once I feel comfortable, I can quite easily talk for England. I could never have been one of those girls that went back to school and was straight away the loudest in the class, but this is ok.

What I want you to remember is that if you are a little shy at first do not worry, because as soon as you feel comfortable with the people around you, I am sure you will be absolutely fine. I was.

Confidence has always been something that has not come easy for me, but I have worked hard on it, especially more recently. I was never any good with groups of people even if I knew them well, but I am now probably one of the loudest in my friendship groups, so things have changed, that is for sure. I still need to work on my confidence when it comes to meeting new people, but these things take time, and there is no rush. Be kind to yourself.

I do not want to give you any fluffy useless advice, as being confident is not just flicking a switch. It takes time like everything else, and you must work at it.

## BULLYING

Bullying, unfortunately, affects many people at some point in their life, just sadly some more than others. I got bullied quite badly in junior school and can still remember it fairly clearly. At that age, it is much harder to deal with hurtful comments. I always struggled more when it came to verbal bullying, as for girls, physical bullying is far less common. My mum would always say "sticks and stones may break your bones, but names will never hurt you" and she was right. Ignoring the bullies is exactly what you should do, and push your emotions aside until you get home. Bullies will only continue if they realise they are affecting you and getting a reaction.

There are two types of bullying: physical bullying and emotional bullying. I have only ever experienced emotional bullying, but that is not to say it is better or worse than physical bullying, as both are awful and something no one should ever have to go through.

Physical Bullying

- Hitting, pushing or knocking you over
- Locking you in or out of rooms/toilets
- Forcing you to do things
- Taking things from you
- Damaging something that belongs to you

Emotional Bullying

- Being threatened
- Getting you into trouble
- Teasing or name calling

- Sending you nasty messages
- Isolating you from your friends and making you feel left out

What can you do if you are being bullied?
From personal experience, bullies will choose someone they are able to gain a reaction from. My advice would be to try as hard as you can to ignore them and ensure they do not succeed with this, however hard it is. Trust me though, it will be worth it if you can hold back the tears until you get home. If you do this enough times, they will get bored and move on.

Another thing to do would be to make a scene in front of people and show them up. They will then most likely stop and not bother you again. Try standing up for yourself, it may take you a while to be able to do this, but once you can, it feels great.

If it is physical bullying, you may want someone to teach you some self-defence. This is generally a useful skill to have in life anyway, just for your own protection in all situations when needed, but please make sure it is for defence only, to protect yourself.

One last thing, talking to a family member, whether it is an older sibling, or your parents, can help you. Someone is likely to have been through something similar, and can therefore give you advice. Whether this helps you or not, a problem shared is a problem halved, and getting it off your chest will feel like a weight has been lifted.

# Mental Health

"NO MATTER HOW YOUR HEART IS GRIEVING, IF YOU KEEP ON BELIEVING, THE DREAM THAT YOU WISH WILL COME TRUE" – *Cinderella*

The term mental health is often mistaken for mental illness. We all have mental health, just like we have physical health, but regardless of whether you have been diagnosed with a mental illness, you have to look after your mental health. Statistics show that 1 in 4 people will experience a mental health problem of some kind each year in England, which shocked me. Mental health awareness is still low, but recently it has gained more funding and awareness than ever before, which is great, but there is still so much we can do to help. You can support mental health campaigns online or in local shops. Donate, fundraise, share your story, engage with others, or volunteer.

## ANXIETY

This is a very personal thing to write about, but if you are reading this as an anxiety sufferer yourself, I hope this will help and support you, and also show you that you are not alone.

Anxiety is such a horrendous feeling and something you often feel you cannot control. There are different levels of anxiety. It may be that going to doctors could be a trigger for you, as personally, that makes me feel all sick inside, or it may be huge crowds of people, both of which are valid reasons. I have always been jealous of those not affected by situations like this, but it could also be past trauma or much larger life experiences that can cause anxiety. High levels of anxiety can also cause panic attacks, whether you are aware of having anxiety or not. The first time I had a panic attack, I had no idea what it was and ended up going to the hospital and spending about 5 hours there. I was terrified, to say the least, and felt like somebody was pushing down on my chest and squeezing my neck.

Not everybody understands anxiety, and that is ok. Even some of the closest people to me do not fully understand it and how it can massively affect someone's day to day life. It is hard, but even if you explain your feelings to someone, they will never truly understand unless they go through it themselves, so just remember this when talking to others, as this can affect their response.

Panic attacks sadly can happen whenever, and in any situation, and they normally last a max of 15-20 minutes but can be longer in severe cases. I am fortunate to experience more general anxiety than panic attacks, but when I have had them in the past, they have not lasted too long, and after becoming more in tune with my body, I can control them a little more. I also find my panic attacks are shorter if I am home and by myself, rather than in public or with anyone, as that only makes it worse when trying to calm myself down.

For me, my anxiety is why I tend not to go to crowded places as I always feel too claustrophobic, and my anxiety is the worst in these situations. I would much rather avoid them and stay at home, or go to my quiet local pub. I am aware that this is something not many people my age do, but I am much happier this way, and that is all that matters. New people and large venues also make me anxious, so when I choose to go to my local pub in the village, it is not because I am lazy or boring, it is because this is my comfort zone and staying within this keeps my anxiety at bay.

What helps me?
Walking away from the situation I am in, whether I am at work, or a social environment, just stepping outside into the fresh air makes a difference.

Slow and deep breaths, trying to focus on your breathing alone and nothing else. If at home, meditation helps me relax and focus on being in the moment. I have found that guided meditation apps and videos have made such a difference to the regularity of my anxiety since taking time to listen to them. Do not force yourself to meditate, but if you can even squeeze in a 5-minute video and just listen while lying on your bed, I can assure you it will do wonders with your mental state at that moment. It may make you cry or want to express a few types of emotions, but this is a good thing and a way of release.

In terms of treatment, I hate going to the doctors, so I put this off for a while, but eventually got the courage to go. I saw a therapist for my depression and anxiety, as well as being prescribed a course of medication, which helped.

Sunlight is also proven to uplift your mood. Getting your daily dose of vitamin D by going outside is great for looking after your mental health.

Just remember you are not alone, and anxiety is extremely common. Do not let this affect your personality and your confidence. Go and see all the places you want to visit, but do not force yourself. Go when you feel ready, and just remember to be happy.

Now, I have a little task for you. If you do the below in pencil or even in a notebook, you can come back to this daily or weekly with a fresh mind.

Write down 3 things you are currently anxious about

1. exams (gcses)

2. my life ahead of me.

3.

Now choose one of them and write 3 things you could do to help the situation

1.

2.

3.

Focusing on one thing at a time really helps clear your mind. I find if there is a lot of anxiety present, it can become far too overwhelming and is far easier to break it down, so that you have the energy and ability to deal with each and every emotion, in your own time.

## DEPRESSION

Another touchy taboo subject, but I do feel depression is something that needs to be spoken about more often, especially with the younger generation.

Personally, I never really knew what depression was until I was 20 years old and lost someone very close to me due to suicide. Having someone close to me suffer from depression helped me to gain an understanding of this illness.

Depression has a wide range of symptoms, and it affects every person differently. You may lose complete interest in any hobbies or things you used to enjoy, feeling worthless and unhappy, as well as emotionally drained and tearful. Symptoms can also be very similar to anxiety, and you may experience physical symptoms too, such as loss of appetite and exhaustion. The severity of the symptoms range from mild to severe, and most of us in our lives will go through periods of feeling upset and down, which is normal. Depression, on the other hand, is that very same feeling, but constantly, for weeks, months, or perhaps even years, and it can make you feel as though continuing with life is pointless.

Depression is not a sign of weakness. The feelings of stress or low mood are common, it just depends how long this lasts for, as to whether this is a sign of depression.

You never know what someone is going through and what battles they may be fighting alone. Message your friends and family today, and tell them what they mean to you. Spread some positivity and love. The power of negative or harmful words and actions can push somebody over the edge, and this is not ok. Think before you speak, before you message, before you comment, and think before you share. Go and create those happy memories instead of making unhappy ones for others. Be kind always, as what you say has a lasting impact.

"In a world where you can be anything, be kind"

- *Caroline Flack*

## WORKING OUT FOR YOUR MENTAL HEALTH

Studies have shown that certain exercises can reduce anxiety or depression. Increasing circulation to the brain has a positive effect on your HPA axis, which is your stress hormone response. This then influences your overall mood. Working out in the morning typically wakes you up, which is why many people choose this to start their day off right. However, I have to be honest, I often could not think of anything worse than a morning workout, but if you can find the motivation, the statement is true, I have to admit, and you will feel far better by doing so. This then sets you up for a deeper sleep in the evenings, meaning you are then getting fit and sleeping better, which in due course will have such a positive impact on your life.

Regular exercise can be a challenging habit to put into place, but once created, the benefits massively outweigh the temptations of going back to your old lazy ways. Get yourself some new cute gym wear as I find this helps with my motivation, and if you can afford to spend that little extra on a luscious gym membership, it makes all the difference.

Movement of any sort, whether this is running, walking, or dancing, moves your lymph and blood flow. Having a healthy lymph flow helps avoid bloating and swelling, as well as preventing the stagnation of toxins in your body so that you can avoid catching a bug, and keep inflammation levels low. An overall win-win situation.

Getting into an exercise routine can be a challenge for some, I know it is for me, that is for sure. Exercise for me has always felt like a chore, something I dislike but have no choice in the matter if I want to keep my body moving and healthy. Not everyone enjoys a hardcore workout, and if that is you, then that is ok, as there are plenty of ways to exercise without feeling like you could pass out at the end, so do not be afraid to try something new as you may completely surprise yourself and enjoy it. I, for one, have recently started adding spinning classes into my routine. Some days I can manage an intense 30-minute cycle, and others, a relaxed 15 minutes is all I feel up to doing, and both are ok.

It honestly does not have to be that bad, perhaps try out a new hobby, pop outside for a nice walk, or get that rusty bike out of the shed. Keeping fit is literally on your doorstep, whether you live in a city or a tiny village like me. Even 10 minutes of exercise a day can really lift your mood and massively help to relieve any stress or anxiety, which in the long run will improve your mental health as well as your physical health.

Having that time to switch off will do you the world of good, but try not to let yourself fall off the exercise wagon due to some little excuse. It is just a matter of finding that form of exercise that works for you, and if this takes time do not worry, as I am nearing 30 and have only just found a form of exercise I enjoy and do not dread the thought of.

Last year I took up dance classes which have had such a positive impact on my life, and I love it. Fantastic for my health and fitness, but also my mental state. It does not have to be anything strenuous or high impact, if it makes you feel good both physically and mentally, then that is all that matters.

## TRAUMA

Trauma is an emotional response to a traumatic event in your life where, immediately after, you are often in shock or denial. Trauma is divided into three main types: Acute, chronic and complex.

Acute trauma mainly results from a single distressing event such as an assault or an accident in which the person's emotional or physical security is threatened, leaving a lasting impression on the person's mind. Often medical help is needed as, if left untreated, it can affect how the person thinks and behaves.

Chronic trauma may occur when a person is exposed to a long-term illness, abuse, bullying, as well as a build-up of several events of acute trauma. Chronic trauma can often take years after the event to show symptoms and often has a severe impact on the person's mind. These individuals may have trust issues and struggle with stability in their lives.

Complex trauma generally refers to events between people, such as relationships. This could include childhood abuse or neglect and affects the person's overall health, relationships, and other aspects of their life.

Trauma. We can heal from it, although it is not easy. We tend to push seemingly less significant smaller traumas aside, but these are still traumas, and the build-up can have everlasting hard-hitting effects on our lives when not dealt with. Some may say give it time, but from my perspective and opinion, I would say getting support and help at the time rather than pushing it aside is needed. Personally, I regret not getting professional support with a few traumatic times in my life.

Support such as group or individual therapy not only allows you to work through past experiences, but also allows you to process ways of dealing with any future traumas you may come across. Professional help will give you the coping mechanisms needed with any future hiccups or traumas, rather than letting them build up, as no matter how strong you are mentally as a person, there is a limit as to how much you can take on.

Throughout life you are bound to experience ups and downs, highs and lows, but when it comes to those low moments, how you handle them is key to a happy life.

## DEALING WITH LOSS

We will all experience loss in our lives at some point, whether this is a family member or friend, and it is one of the toughest things we ever have to go through. I was fortunate to have both sets of grandparents throughout my entire childhood, so I never had to experience the death of a loved one until I was 20, when I lost a boyfriend of mine through suicide. The percentage of deaths through suicide is increasing yearly, but you never think it would happen to anyone you know, and if I am honest, at the time, it felt like my world had ended. It was the hardest thing I have ever had to go through, and hugely upsetting to realise there are people out there that would prefer to not be in this world at all, which massively pulled on my heartstrings.

I then lost two grandparents, and my great-grandma within a short space of time. My grandparents have all played a huge part in my life growing up and losing two of them affected me more than I could have imagined. One of the closest people to me in my life is my grandma, and I honestly am dreading the day she is no longer here as she means so much to me.

Even to this day, I think about those I have lost in my life, daily. It is ok to think about them, and there is no shame in this, as memories are an important part of life. Do not let these thoughts stop you from moving on and enjoying your own life though, as you know they would only want the best for you, and not for you to be held back because of them.

Therapy should be an option to consider if you feel you are struggling. Having someone to talk to about your grief in an honest but confidential way, means you can express your true feelings without any judgement.

Therapists are there to listen so that you have someone as a support that can hold you up, so to speak, and is emotionally stable to take it, but can also help advise you with ways of coping. Having coping mechanisms and finding ways that help you are so important, as we are all different, and the way your friend deals with loss may be the complete opposite of what helps you.

## INNER CRITIC

The world and our thoughts have become so accustomed to negative self-talk. Having that little voice in your head daily, telling you things such as you are ugly or you are stupid, even from a young age can be detrimental. Most of us would not dream of saying those things to our friends and family, so why do we feel it is acceptable to say these things to ourselves?

I have recently become far more aware of the things I say or think, and how I put myself down far too often when we can do anything we set our minds to. Having awareness of why you may be having these negative thoughts about yourself, whatever it is regarding, is the foundation for changing how you may feel.

Exploring the reasons, whether this is a past comment from someone you love or a childhood event, will truly help you fight your inner critic.

Sadly, it can often only take that one negative comment for your confidence and belief in yourself to decrease, and for you to give up, or perhaps not even start.

Another reason could be an experience, maybe you tried something as a child and struggled, so it made you feel you cannot do it, even though we evolve and change so much in our lives, meaning you should always give everything a second chance. I used to think I could not cook in the slightest and I know you are probably thinking what has this got to do with anything, but trust me, I lived off ready meals for years, thinking I cannot cook so why bother. Anyway, it turns out, I can cook and have had friends request my tuna pasta bake recipe, as even they cannot make it as delicious as mine. Something simple I know, but we all start somewhere and need to give ourselves credit for even the little things in life.

Another example for you. I, like most young girls, tried dance when I was little and had no coordination and struggled to even move in time with the music. Last year however, I tried dance classes again, and can now do it without even thinking. We all start somewhere and even if you fail the first time, do not let this make you give up. You are capable of anything you set your mind to. Remember that.

## BE KIND TO YOURSELF

Just a reminder, if the weekend is coming up, or it is mid-week and you have an evening without any plans, schedule some time to rest.

Whether that is sitting in a comfy spot and reading a book or listening to music, do something relaxing for your mind and look after yourself. Switch off all screens and focus on a little bit of "you time". This helps reset the body and mind when things are getting a little too much.

Journaling is another fantastic release of emotions. Get yourself a new pretty notebook, and each evening, write down exactly how you felt that day, whatever the emotions. Write them all down, just make sure afterwards that you end on three positives from the day, or things you are grateful for, as this means you end your evening on a positive note and your mind goes to sleep happy.

There is a lot going on in the world, and even for me personally, I have been so up and down mentally. I can feel on top of the world one minute, and the next I could just cry. If you are feeling the same, do not be so hard on yourself, as every single one of us has days like these, and you would not be normal without them. Putting time aside to focus on yourself is the most important thing in life. How can you love someone if you cannot love yourself?

Perhaps try a new sport or craft, something to take your mind off things, or even just going out for a short walk can have such a huge impact on your day. Just five minutes in the fresh air without your phone or any distractions can help try and reset how you are feeling, just remember that life only throws things at you that you can handle.

You can do this, you can get through this, you just need to believe in yourself.

Write down 3 things you are grateful for today.

1.

2.

3.

# Happiness

"THINK HAPPY THOUGHTS" -*Peter Pan*

## YOUR PERSONAL SPACE

Finding that personal space where you can feel yourself and relax, is so important. I, for one, do not have to worry about finding that space as I live alone, but for those living at home with parents still, maybe yours would be your bedroom. The most important thing is to ensure you feel completely relaxed in your surroundings. If my place is clean and tidy, it makes such a difference to my mental state.

Having everything organised is also another big thing for me, as I dislike clutter, and am very minimalistic with my decor, but obviously, everyone is different. I also love neutral earthy colours and find these very calming, but if bright colours are what tickles your fancy, then totally go for it.

## INTERNET DETOX

This is something I never in a million years thought I would do, or even think about, but for world mental health day, I decided to stop any form of messaging and social media for a whole 24 hours. If I am being completely honest, it was one of the best things I have ever done. Listening to my body and mind by doing what I want to do for a day, rather than spending most of the day on my phone, scrolling through apps looking at what others are getting up to. It is easier said than done, I must admit, but I truly realised how important real life is, and that living life through your phone is making what used to be normal life, now a distant memory for some people.

Going on walks, having a coffee catch up, or even reading a book, are all things we keep pushing aside and not making time for, due to our screens. It may be a little excessive to put your phone aside for a whole day like I did, but if you could even do an hour, it will make a world of difference to your life. Doing a digital detox gives your mind that chance to switch off and focus on the things that matter in life without digital distraction.

Spending too much time on the internet can be seriously detrimental to your mental health, and you can end up feeling disconnected from reality. I get carried away and do not realise how long I am spending on my phone each day until I check my screen time and am in complete shock.

So, for those of you that are like me, maybe scheduling some screen-free time each day, is the best way forward. That way, you can be totally in control. If you struggle to limit your screen time, you can set up limits and downtime using settings on your phone. I find the first and last thing I do each day is to check my phone, so maybe have the first and last hour each day, to relax, read a book, or start journaling. Ask yourself why you are scrolling through social media for so long each day and what the positives are for doing this, and if you do not find any, then perhaps it is time to re-evaluate. Take control and feel completely free to press that unfollow button if you are scrolling through and various posts are not bringing you any joy. I have stuck to having some time off each week from my phone and am loving it.

An entire day spent without social media when I spend every day scrolling through platforms, posting and sharing was going to be a challenge, but the results were incredible and massively worth it. I spent the day caring and focusing on myself rather than other people's lives on Instagram that have no relevance. I still found myself picking up my phone a lot, which made me realise how much I relied on it and how it is such a big part of my life. The whole day I had that feeling at the back of my mind that I was missing out, when in fact, being on my phone as much as I am, means I miss out on so much daily. Think of all the things you could do instead of all that wasted time scrolling.

Since then, my time has been spent so differently. I have added a list of interests to my life, and my mental health has improved because of this.

Finally, stop comparing yourself to others. What you see on social media platforms are the edited highlights of people's lives, remember this.

## HEALTH

Your health, whether you realise it or not, plays a part in your everyday happiness. I noticed recently that I was feeling incredibly tired during the day, and this was affecting my work ethic as well as my health. I was going to bed far too late, watching television for hours and then having to get up early for work. Totalling around five hours of sleep is not enough for your body to function properly. Diet also plays a huge part. I noticed I was eating whenever I wanted, and more often than not, I was choosing unhealthy options. Your body, to survive and for your organs to be healthy, needs a balanced diet, or you will experience various changes as well as consequences to your health.

Drinking plenty of water and avoiding sugary drinks will also be very beneficial to your health and your happiness. Treat your body how you would treat any other living thing. You would feed your pet what it needs rather than what it wants, so make sure you do this for yourself too. I understand that changing your dietary habits can be challenging, as who would choose a salad over a burger, let's be honest, but ensuring you keep that balance is important.

Regular medical checkups are also key. When it comes to any health issues, big or small, it is best to keep on top of things so that you can treat any issues early. I have regular blood tests, and was recently advised I am anaemic and was put on iron tablets, but without this checkup, I would be none the wiser.

## THERAPY

This is something I never thought I would need. No one feels they will end up needing therapy in their life, but quite honestly, it changed my life. I had therapy for the first time when I was 20 years old after losing my dear friend Samuel.

What I will say, is that no matter whether you think your life is great or not, everyone should take some time for therapy sessions in their schedule. It changes how you see life.

Most people think therapy is for those going through severe depression, and that it is that final resort to pull themselves out, but why not have therapy so that you can keep on top of your life and everything going on so that you do not end up lowering yourself into that depressive frame of mind and end up using it as a final resort.

I have found friends to be hugely supportive whenever I am having one of those days, but they will always have their own opinions on anything you mention to them, and their own problems to deal with. Therapists, on the other hand, are there purely to listen to you, without any judgement. They are there to offer advice if needed, but can also just be there for you to sit and talk to for an hour, let your emotions out, and then leave feeling refreshed with a weight lifted off your shoulders. Therapy is nothing to be afraid of as they only have your best interests at heart and are purely there to help.

Lots of things happen in our lives that we cannot control, and these things will leave us feeling a wide range of emotions. Whether these are big or small, we will keep these thoughts with us until we have processed them and are able to let go. Things that happen over the years tend to build up, and then one day when you least expect it, all these emotions will hit you at once and this is called a mental breakdown. By going to therapy, you can avoid all these pressures building up and causing large amounts of upset.

## MEDITATION

This is a recent discovery for me, and something until this year I had never thought about even trying. I saw it as a pointless thing to do and did not see how it could benefit anyone's life, but how wrong and mistaken I was. During a habits course I took part in recently, we discussed ways of adding things into our lives that would only benefit us, and this is where meditation comes in. It was in one of the sessions within the course, that I tried meditation for the first time, and I cried.

It turns out that meditation often gives you what you need at that particular time, which that day for me, was to let out some emotions. Since then, meditation has been a huge part of my life and pretty much part of my daily routine. This has meant a few more tears, but also extra sleep. It is so incredible that as I am writing this now, I am thinking about which guided meditation I want to do next.

Meditation means rather than dwelling over the past or worrying about the future, it encourages you to remain in the moment and become aware of your current emotions to achieve a mentally and emotionally clear and stable state.

During meditation, your mind may wander, and that is ok and part of the wonderful experience of letting go and trusting the process of your emotions. The journey is more important than the destination and the time it takes to get there. It takes time to become comfortable with your emotions, and I, for one, am a professional when it comes to pushing my feelings aside and just continuing with my daily life, but this will not benefit you. There may be some setbacks, but you can overcome these. You are doing great. When you first start meditation, you may feel a little overwhelmed, and this is normal.

You can meditate pretty much anywhere, but preferably somewhere quiet where you can close your eyes and listen to every breath as you slowly breathe in and out. Meditation is not about stopping your thoughts but about observing your emotions and developing awareness.

Deciding on the time and place that suits you is the first step. Research shows that it is easier to form a habit when adding something new into your routine, and to meditate at the same place and time each day. When you first begin to meditate, I would suggest starting with manageable amounts of time so that it is achievable. Putting too much pressure on yourself from the start will only make the habit less easy to maintain, and you can always build it up. Making sure you find a comfortable place to lie down or sit before you start, is key. I find lying on top of the duvet on my bed, or the floor is best for me, but I know my mum, for example, prefers the hard kitchen floor, so it is completely up to you. It is best if your back is straight and your body is relaxed.

There are different forms of meditation, but when starting, I would suggest a guided meditation, as this is led by an experienced teacher, and all you have to do is listen. I tend to choose 10-minute long sessions, but some can last up to an hour.

You will most likely already be familiar with the amount of benefits meditation can bring to your life when it comes to your mental health, but it is important to realise the physical effects it can have on your body too. Stress stimulates the sympathetic nervous system, which as a result can negatively impact the body by causing stress hormones in the bloodstream, which can increase the risks of heart attacks. Too much cortisol, which is a stress hormone, can increase blood sugar levels and also affect your immune system. Meditation helps because when your mind and body are relaxed, your stress hormones are no longer stimulated and released into the bloodstream. You will also notice your blood pressure levels will decrease, and your sleep will increase, if you are less stressed. It can also decrease negative neurological connections to the medial prefrontal cortex of the brain, as well as increasing the cortical thickness, which is responsible for memory and learning, and so therefore a thicker cortex through the practice of meditation will help with emotional regulation.

## MINDFULNESS

Mindfulness is a form of meditation in which you focus on being intensely aware and present at that moment. Setting time aside for mindfulness each day is so important. Listen and be mindful of your body and what it needs.

This can be used in physical situations such as your exercise routine, or it can be used when it comes to your eating schedule, both of which are just as important. It is all about being present and aware of what your body needs and not overdoing it or forcing yourself to do something your body does not want. Often our food and exercise routines are not mindful.

When we are mindful, we enhance our awareness and increase our attention to our well-being, reducing stress by approaching the situation with kindness and paying attention to our thoughts without any judgement. Reminding ourselves that there is no should or should not, right or wrong way to think or feel. It is about acknowledging and accepting our thoughts and feelings at that given moment. It is easy to get caught up in our feelings and try and correct ourselves, without stopping to notice our true emotions and how our thoughts are driving our behaviours. When we are truly in touch with our bodies and how we feel, we can change how we see ourselves and our lives for the better.

## JOURNALING

Research shows that those who journal had an increase in performance compared to those who did not. It is one of the most effective ways to reduce stress. Writing in detail about your emotions and feelings is a form of release. It is a chance for you to reflect and work on any current problems you may have, whether this is a recent upset or a past trauma, instead of keeping everything locked away and potentially letting it build up and cause more damage. It is a way of expressing your emotions, and I find the old-fashioned notebook and pen method works well for this.

As well as a de-stress in the current moment, it is also something great for looking back on and a way of tracking your personal growth.

The pages you write are for your eyes only, so write down your exact thoughts and emotions at that moment and do not hold back, as the more honest with yourself you can be, the more you will gain from the experience.

As much as journaling is good if you have had a stressful or upsetting day, it does not always have to be something you do when you have unwanted emotions. It can also be for those happy ones, such as writing the things you are grateful for that day.

Journaling can be a form of therapy or to offload. Writing allows you to process anything you may be struggling with and can often lead to problem-solving. I often journal about past trauma of mine and find writing things down helps me. It is all about finding beneficial coping mechanisms that work for you.

Growing up I would always push anything I found challenging to deal with to one side and escape from it rather than face it and learn from it, but since then I have introduced journaling into my life as well as therapy, and have found they go well hand in hand, and my past trauma is not seeming as heavy anymore. Do not get me wrong, the change does not happen overnight, but if you journal regularly, it should not take long until you feel a weight being lifted.

I started a blog around three years ago, and I did not realise it, but this is actually a form of journaling. I have always blogged about rather personal topics and found that the days I blogged ended up being the days I felt the lightest. I always wondered why and only realised recently that I was releasing emotions within my posts and that it was benefiting me mentally by doing so. You do not have to make it public if you would prefer not to, but it is nice to look back and see how far you have come. Helping people has always been so important to me, and it helps my mental state, as the focus is on others rather than myself. Talking about the past, however traumatic some of it may be, helps process it and move on, as pushing any traumatic event aside will only do more harm than good to you mentally.

## GRATITUDE

With gratitude, we acknowledge the goodness in our lives. It helps us to feel positive emotions, relish good experiences, and improve our health and well-being.

Gratitude from the Latin word gratus is a feeling of appreciation. The benefits are endless, and those who regularly take time to reflect upon the things they are grateful for are known to feel more in touch with themselves and their feelings, sleep better, express more kindness, as well as experience positive emotions more often. If you are anything like me, you may be more motivated to watch Netflix and go on your phone, than write in your journal and practice gratitude. Noticing new things you are grateful for each day works, and while you might be thankful for things such as your family and your health, noticing the smaller things such as having a few minutes for a cup of tea in silence, keeps your brain alert for fresh moments to journal.

It is proven that those who wrote gratitude lists compared to those who wrote about negative experiences, reported significantly better mental health. This suggests gratitude writing can be beneficial for not only those that are healthy mentally but also for those that struggle with their mental health. This works by shifting those negative thoughts into positive ones and bringing your attention away from toxic emotions. It is important to note that these shifts take time when it comes to the benefits of gratitude writing, but practicing the experience of gratitude could overall contribute to improved mental health over time. Most of our energy is spent focusing on those things we do not currently have, whereas gratitude helps us prioritise and learn to appreciate the things we do have.

Celebrating your accomplishments, even if it is something small like making your bed in the morning, can retrain your brain and allow you to appreciate those positive thoughts.

## MANIFESTING

If you think it, it will come. Manifestation is essentially bringing your thoughts to life, however, there is more to it. As I have said before, things do not happen overnight, and even though manifestation is about turning those dreams into reality, you still have to work for it.

First off, you need to know what you want as you are the only one who dreams your dreams. The next step is to create your visualisation, whether this is by saying it out loud, writing it down, or through meditation. You may also be familiar with the 369 method, where you write down what you want in the following order: 3 times in the morning, 6 times in the afternoon, and 9 times at night, which I find magical. Just always remember when going through this process, to be mindful and grateful for what you already have, or will receive.

The Law of Attraction suggests that positive thoughts bring positive outcomes, and the same goes for negative thoughts. What you focus on is what you draw into your life, creating your reality. Having a more optimistic outlook on life may help you stay motivated to work towards your goals and dreams.

Life is a blank canvas, and you are in control of what goes on it. Creating pictures of our intended life, and then using choices to make this reality. If you often have days where you struggle to be in a positive mindset, perhaps try setting yourself small daily goals that can build up over time, such as engaging in positive self-talk each day. As a result, by changing our self-talk and how we feel about life, we reverse the negative patterns and form more positive, healthy, and productive ones. One good thing leads to another, and the direction of a life can shift from a downward spiral to an upward ascent. There are some exercises such as journaling, positive self-talk, or creating your very own mood board that can help you to put the Law of Attraction into place in your own life.

## FORWARD PLANNING

Making goals for yourself is such a great way of taking positive control of your own life. The past year I have just been plodding along as normal and not stopping to think that all these hours, days, and months are going past, and I do not have any form of direction. I am such a planner with everything else in my life, and I have a passion for organising, but things such as yearly plans had not even crossed my mind, and when mentioned, just seemed daunting. I then came to realise, there do not have to be massive changes in my life or big plans, but even something small such as planning gym sessions or adding a new hobby into my week, or perhaps even making time to read my book, would add such positivity to my life.

Structure has such a positive impact on your brain and how you function. I use a calendar app on my phone to plan out my weeks with time slots, making myself feel organised and that I have my life together, even if it is like I say, the little things. Start with weekly plans and organising each day until you feel comfortable moving on to planning the months or years ahead.

## HABITS

Habits are things you do on a daily or weekly basis that can be either beneficial to your life or not. Small decisions and actions you perform every day. Habits start with a psychological pattern called a habit loop, a process with three parts: the cue, routine and reward. The cue is something that perhaps triggers you to undertake a task, the routine is the behaviour itself, whether this is emotional, physical or mental, and the reward is what you gain. This then gives you the motivation, and stimulates you to remember this in the future, causing this to then be a habit.

I would recommend getting a notebook and writing down the things you do daily, and working out whether these are beneficial to your life or not. Perhaps you are like me and each morning when you wake up, the first thing you do is check your phone? Even if I do not have any notifications, I find myself scrolling endlessly through social media, checking each platform both morning and evening in bed, when perhaps I could be doing something that benefits my life, even if this is just reading my book during these times instead. I snooze my alarm numerous times each morning as I lack the motivation to get out of bed and would much rather sleep. But those few minutes extra in bed will most likely only make you feel more tired, so try putting your phone on the other side of your room before you fall asleep so that when your alarm goes off in the morning, you physically have to get out of bed to turn it off. Getting up and out of bed, even for an alarm will make such a difference, and you will then find you are ready to start your day.

To change the habits that perhaps do not benefit your life, you need to want to change, but once you start the process you will find other unhealthy habits will also fade away alongside the habits you are focusing on, and it becomes natural.

Exercising is one of the best things you can do first thing in the morning. It gives you that adrenaline rush, then with a shower and a healthy breakfast afterwards, you will feel full of energy to go about your day, but I understand the motivation to get up and do this can be a struggle. I have lost count of the number of times I have set an alarm for 6 or 7 in the morning to do a quick workout before starting work, and have ended up staying in bed instead. I have even set up my laptop with an online workout loaded ready and put out my clothes so that I only have to press play and get dressed, but even that did not work. It is not easy, but most things in life can be a challenge if done right.

There are going to be many times in your life where things can be a struggle and you may feel slightly overwhelmed and as if you cannot achieve what it is you are trying to do, but this is not a reason to give up. Not one single person in this world achieves something big overnight, but it can be done by creating small new habits that you can add to your daily or weekly life, to make stepping stones to achieve your end goal.

Habits are all about creating those little daily tasks so that the larger task or goal does not seem so big and overwhelming.

Speak nicely to yourself. I had never noticed the way I speak unkindly to myself until this was pointed out to me recently. If you fail to achieve something, you may notice you criticise yourself, whether this is out loud or in your head. All these things will only help your mind think you cannot do it. Rather than saying something negative, try giving yourself a positive boost. Shaking your body all over to give yourself a mini reset and saying motivational words to yourself with a positive action, for example jumping in the air, will put you in that mindset to achieve. This is something I learnt in my dance classes that has stuck with me.

Tell yourself you can, rather than you cannot. You can do anything your mind sets itself to do.

Acknowledging what you are grateful for is another fantastic motivational habit to include in your daily routine. Waking up feeling positive each morning and writing down three things that you are grateful for can have a huge impact on how your day will go. Have you ever woken up in a foul mood and remained that way for the rest of the day or perhaps even longer? You can avoid this by choosing a positive mindset the minute you wake up, and listing the things you are happy about, grateful for, and thinking about those you love. Focusing on a few things you are grateful for is perfect for self-development and you can even set aside a pretty notebook specifically for this. Being able to look back will show how far you have come, and each day you write the things you are grateful for, it will become easier and you will not feel the need to dig as deep as they will be on the surface.

Be around positive people. Your friendships should encourage you and lift you, and if you are not getting that in a friendship, then you should reconsider it. The people that feel like bright blue skies, these are the ones you need in your life. It took me years to figure this out and I wish someone had told me this when I was growing up. You cannot change or choose your family, but you have the right to change and choose your friends, so choose wisely. I am fortunate to have a handful of incredible, life-changing, supportive, happy friends, some of which have been in my life since I was young, and I am so grateful for every one of them.

Putting yourself first is also so important. Do not feel you have to say yes to everything. You need to sometimes stop trying to please everyone, and instead, just sit back, relax, and focus on what you want to be doing. This is not selfish at all. If you do not feel like going out and meeting a friend this week, then you do not have to. You cannot always neglect your own needs for others.

At the start of the year, I completed a self-development course over Zoom which has changed my perception of various things in my life. I have been working since then, on changing habits and implementing positive changes into my daily routine. Quite often we cannot recognise the difference between habits that benefit our lives, and ones that do not.

The course was a little tough mentally for me but only because we discussed topics that may, for some people, bring up past trauma or any current issues. This is a good thing though, as speaking openly about topics you find challenging, is a way of coping, which then brings positive changes to your life and that is incredible. Hearing other people's stories within the group on the course helped me, and knowing I was not alone, as quite often we become quite isolated with our thoughts until someone speaks up and we then realise we are not the only one. It has been inspiring and rather life-changing for me though, as there were quite a few unhealthy habits I wanted to remove from my daily life that were causing a negative effect, and I have already made small changes to these. I have also learnt little techniques and tips to add certain things into my routine to benefit me.

You should be proud of yourself and how far you have come. Do not ever change yourself for someone else. You are you, and you are enough.

## SLEEP

Sleep is something we all need, to be able to function, but various things can affect the amount of sleep you get each night. I am sure I am not alone when I say I am on my phone a lot in the evening, but without us fully even realising, being on your phone can disrupt your sleep pattern. Perhaps try putting your phone aside an hour before you want to sleep. Read a book, meditate, or even journal. Both your phone and television screens can help keep you awake as your brain is not able to use this time to switch off. Most phones have a setting that will set your phone to "do not disturb" at the time you tell it to, to help you put your phone aside with enough time for some self-care or relaxation before you sleep.

We often do not realise it, but our last thought before bed can affect how well we sleep, and also any dreams we have. Adding journaling and gratitude lists into your evening routine helps change your thought processes before sleep.

Good sleep is the foundation for good health and a happier mind, but it is easier said than done. Winding down in the evening for at least an hour before you plan on going to sleep is the best remedy for a restful night's sleep. There are hacks you can use to ensure you get the sleep your body needs. Sticking to a routine and going to bed around the same time each day works when it comes to training your mind and body with consistency. You will be surprised by the positive effects that keeping to fixed lights out time each evening can have on your body, as we follow a circadian rhythm that requires a routine.

Time looking at screens such as the television or your phone before bed keeps your mind active and awake and does not give your body time to switch off. I recently discovered the nighttime setting on my phone, which has been a miracle when it comes to falling asleep earlier. You choose the time to sleep and wake up, and it then notifies you 30 minutes beforehand so that you have time to get ready to settle down for the night. No distractions keeping your mind awake, meaning you are likely to have a longer, deeper sleep and feel better for it in the morning. I have noticed after a few small changes to my routine, that the amount of alarms needed to get me up and out of bed in the morning has decreased and this is a huge shift for me which I am proud of.

Waking up refreshed and energised naturally prepares you for a productive positive day, whereas you may notice if you wake up tired, the chances of that happening are not as great and you may not make those wise decisions. Tiredness can have negative effects on things such as your diet too, and it will become harder to make healthy food choices as your brain loses executive function, meaning that eating a chocolate bar is a go-to option rather than something that would get a nutritionist's approval.

Your bedroom should be a sleep sanctuary: stress and distraction-free. It is proven that the darker the room the better, and having that space for peace is crucial. Some may find listening to some type of ambient sound like white noise can help disrupt any unwanted sounds if you perhaps live in a busy city with traffic noise. Studies have also shown that those surrounded by clutter were more likely to have a sleep disorder, so perhaps listen when your parents say to tidy your room, as a tidy room is a tidy mind and that is the foundation of a good night's sleep. Try meditation to settle the mind, making sure you wind down before you sleep. Lack of sleep can cause knock-on effects on your health and well-being.

Those that struggle with sleep often find they struggle with their mental health as there seems to be a link. This is where remaining mindful at the time of sleep can help relax your mind so that your thoughts do not drift off to thinking about the past or future, causing upset, which is easily done. Meditation or even soothing music is designed to produce a relaxing atmosphere to let your body and mind drift off pleasantly. When it comes to the morning, you can either wake up feeling energised, or you could feel the complete opposite depending on whether you are naturally a morning person or not. If you struggle with your sleep and you do not feel refreshed when you wake, you may find it challenging to drag yourself out of bed, I know I sure do, but learning how to sleep better and creating those healthy habits and routines can help change the feelings when you awake.

Sleep inertia is the transition everyone goes through when adjusting themselves from being asleep to being awake. How much sleep inertia you experience depends on your circadian rhythm, your sleep routine and your habits. Your circadian rhythm is an internal natural process, part of the body's internal clock that runs on a 24-hour cycle. The term circadian comes from the Latin phrase Circa Diem, meaning around a day. When we talk about the circadian rhythm, it is mostly in reference to our sleep cycle, as it aligns our sleep and wakefulness to create a stable cycle of restorative rest, enabling increased daytime activity. At night the signals initiate the production of melatonin which promotes sleep, then in the day, the exposure to light causes the signals to generate alertness instead. If you disturb the sleep-wake circadian rhythm, it can have a lasting effect on your internal body clock, meaning your sleep, as well as your mental and physical health, will be troubled.

## SELF-CARE

Looking after yourself, however selfish it may sound, should be the most important focus in your life.

Waking up in the morning and asking yourself how you are feeling and what you need today, before asking others how they are doing, should be a priority.

Self-care is not instant; it can take work and time to create that happiness. It is not always going to be easy, we all have our bad days, but it will be worth it. They say investing in your mental health should be your first and most focused investment.

Self-care does not mean your focus is purely on positive emotions. Allowing yourself to feel the exact emotion your body needs at that particular time, even if this is negative, will benefit you in the long run.

Dealing with your emotions can often be challenging, but giving yourself time without putting pressure on yourself is so important. A person that is happy all the time does not exist, and fake happiness is not good for your soul. Let yourself experience different emotions, from happy, to sad, or even angry. You do not have to be happy and positive all the time, no one is, just make sure the negative emotions are slightly controlled and not too regular.

Stepping away from situations, perhaps having a social media break, or going for a nice long walk or run can help the process. Techniques and different lifestyle changes can help to manage your mental health and may prevent the need for treatment, although please note that if you are suffering from your mental health, sadly even dramatic positive changes to your life may not resolve the issues, especially if it is past trauma, and you may need a professional's help.

Feeling confident and comfortable with yourself takes time. There is not a single person in this world that does not take anything to heart, but if you can avoid reacting to messages, thoughts or comments, it will help reset your mindset.

Having that basic routine, including daily hygiene, will have a massive impact on how you view life. Brush your teeth, shower, and brush your hair, even when times are tough, as looking after your hygiene is one of the first things to slack, when your mental health is affected.

## SELF-LOVE

Some say love makes the world go round, others describe love as painful because if not returned, it can cause heartache.

We hear about love all the time, but self-love is not discussed as often as it should be. Self-love is the foundation of a healthy life. To start that journey of self-love, we must implement healthy habits into our everyday life. Having a routine that works for you is so important.

Try looking into a mirror, making eye contact with yourself and saying powerful positive thoughts. This is something I never thought of doing until I had a private dance session, and my teacher told me to look at myself in the mirror and say positive words to myself. This I hated, as it was completely out of my comfort zone and something I had not done before, but I appreciated being introduced to this, as it is something I still do now, and feel over time it has helped me. Those who love themselves can express self-love without the feeling of embarrassment, but understandably, this takes time. Try this once a day, using the below phrases as examples, and see how you feel after a week.

- I am strong and powerful
- I am beautiful
- I can do this

Self-love does not come overnight and is something you need to work hard on, but only when you are emotionally ready will you be able to love yourself.

Many of us have past traumas we never dealt with, so often focusing on the past is the best way to then prepare your present and future self. Advice from those around you can massively help, or perhaps you could try an outsiders opinion and see a therapist, but at the end of the day, self-love is deep within and only you can reach it when you are ready.

# My Thoughts Journal

“IF YOU CAN DREAM IT, YOU CAN DO IT” -*Walt Disney*

A journal to change your life like I have changed mine. Reframe those thoughts of yours into positive ones to choose happiness.

## YOU ARE YOU

How would you describe yourself?

1.

2.

3.

4.

5.

6.

7.

8.

Things you love about yourself.

1.

2.

3.

4.

5.

6.

7.

8.

Your best personality traits are.

1.

2.

3.

4.

5.

6.

7.

8.

# YOUR LIFE IS YOURS

What do you want to change?

How are you feeling about this?

What are you going to do to make these changes?

# TODAY IS YOUR DAY

What are you worried about?

What are your thoughts about the situation?

How will you cope with this?

How do you feel now?

What would be your advice to a friend if they had these thoughts?

What self-care are you going to do today?

Who can you turn to when you worry?

1.

2.

3.

4.

5.

What are your favourite things for when life gets overwhelming?

1.

2.

3.

4.

5.

What are your favourite happy movies?

1.

2.

3.

4.

5.

**ABOUT YOU**

Your favourite songs currently.

1. ______________________________

2. ______________________________

3. ______________________________

4. ______________________________

5. ______________________________

The people that inspire you the most.

1.

2.

3.

4.

5.

What makes you happy?

1.

2.

3.

4.

5.

6.

7.

8.

What are you grateful for this year so far?

1.

2.

3.

4.

5.

6.

7.

8.

What are 4 things that you want to achieve next year?

1.

2.

3.

4.

What are 4 things you want to achieve over the next 5 years?

1.

2.

3.

4.

Your reading list.

1.

2.

3.

4.

5.

## BUCKET LIST

1. 

2. 

3. 

4. 

5. 

6.

7.

8.

9.

10.

11.

12.

13.

14.

15.

16.

17.

18.

19.

20.

## GRATEFUL LOVING

### January

I am grateful for

1.

2.

3.

**February**

I am grateful for

1.

2.

3.

**March**

I am grateful for

1.

2.

3.

**April**

I am grateful for

1.

2.

3.

**May**

I am grateful for

1.

2.

3.

**June**

I am grateful for

1.

2.

3.

**July**

I am grateful for

1.

2.

3.

**August**

I am grateful for

1.

2.

3.

**September**

I am grateful for

1.

2.

3.

**October**

I am grateful for

1.

2.

3.

**November**

I am grateful for

1.

2.

3.

**December**

I am grateful for

1.

2.

3.

Change does not happen overnight, but growth is massively important for a happy, healthy life. If you have taken some time to fill in this journal, even if it is only a few words, I am proud of you for taking those first steps, and you should be too.

Keep focusing on you. You are doing great.

## MY HAPPY PLAYLIST

Just thought I would end on a massively positive note, and provide you with my happy playlist. I find whenever I am having a down moment, or I need to focus on positive thoughts rather than letting my mind wander, I simply Bluetooth my phone to a speaker and blast out these songs. Everybody needs songs in their life that instantly boosts their mood, and sharing mine in the hope that they boost yours, makes me feel happy. Music is great for your soul and health.

One For The Road - Nathan Carter

Confetti - Little Mix

Go Down Deh - Spice, Shaggy, Sean Paul

Twist And Shout - The Beatles

Reach - S Club 7

Hillbilly Rock - Johnny Brady

Bruises - Train

Life Is Worth Living - Justin Bieber

One Too Many - Keith Urban, P!nk

Good Time - Niko Moon

Don't Rush - Young T & Bugsey, Headie One

Jenny from the Block - Jennifer Lopez

Havin a Party - Jake Carter

Paper Rings - Taylor Swift

Sarah Jane - Nathan Carter

Pon de Replay - Rihanna

Watermelon Sugar - Harry Styles

Dance with Me Tonight - Olly Murs

Rewrite The Stars - Zak Efron, Zendaya

Let's Get Loud - Jennifer Lopez

Make Believe - Nora Mac

Summer's Here - Nathan Carter

Bad Habits - Ed Sheeran

I Love the Way - Freya Skye

I am no medical expert or professional, and of course nobody is perfect, but I hope I have helped you to become a better and happier version of yourself.

If you do have any questions, or would just like a chat, feel free to send me a message.

Instagram
@annabelletalks

Email
annabelletalks@outlook.com

YouTube
Annabelletalks

Sending you all the love and support on your own wonderful life journey.